RAPID WEIGHT LOSS HYPNOSIS FOR WOMEN

HOW TO LOSE WEIGHT QUICKLY WITH MEDITATION AND AFFIRMATIONS TO INCREASE YOUR SELF-ESTEEM. HEAL YOUR BODY STEP BY STEP WITH APPROPRIATE PSYCHOLOGY.

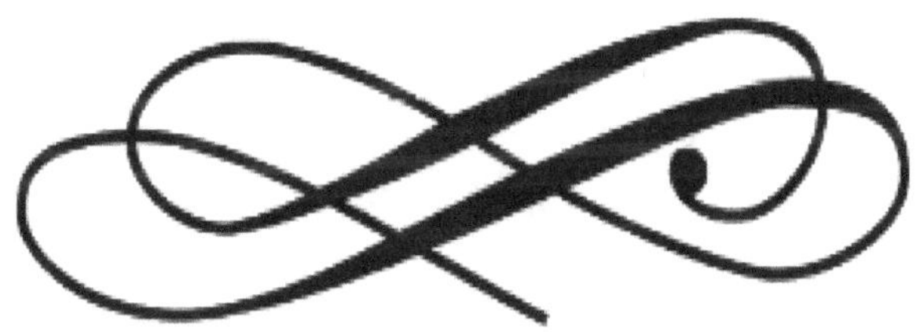

Eva Ruell

© Copyright 2020 - All rights reserved.

Table Of Contents

Introduction

Have you ever wished there was a means to give up smoking or eliminate weight forever and readily? Have you ever had difficulty sleeping and wanted that there was a direct answer? Have you ever wished you could unwind and have more significant memory retention while taking a check? Have you heard of having an ideal connection, being wealthy, and even with good wellness? While these are some pretty amazing objectives, this publication can help you take action in this way.

All of the information which you will need to unwind, restore your wellbeing, remove pain, or become capable of any of your needs is already inside you. This publication will show you how you can discover and use that magic strength, which lies dormant deep inside. All hypnosis is self-hypnosis. You devote nearly all your life to a hypnotizable state.

The definition of hypnosis is only open to tip. You're either free to advise or not. You accept matters, or you refuse them. If you're receptive to suggestions, you're in a more hypnotizable state. That's the foundation of communicating. The further you take and are amenable to tip, the more profound in hypnosis you're. You're being given hints always in almost every area you go and all that you do. This book is going to teach you how you can become mindful of many kinds of proposals you're being bombarded with daily. It occurs everywhere, in your grocery store, restaurants, on T.V. and any kind of media, on the job, while driving, in college, into the family, faith, nightclubs, the authorities, and practically everything else which you take part in.

As soon as you have become conscious of what's occurring, after that, you can take control of everything you reject or accept. You'll have the ability to use the knowledge of self-hypnosis to provide suggestions to advance in attaining your objectives. You are going to learn many strategies to hypnotize yourself permanently and quickly. A lot of these you are most likely doing at this time and are simply unaware of. You are going to learn the myths and roadblocks about alcoholism and also how to prevent them.

You'll have the ability to state your thought process to program yourself for success in each field of life, such as health, prosperity, relationships, joy, and a lot of other subjects. Simply take some opportunity to examine this book and follow the directions given. You may find that upon the conclusion of the book, you won't just have the capability to change just about any area of your life for the higher. Still, you are also going to be in a position to do precisely the same for the lives of your loved ones, friends, and nearest and dearest.

It's best to do this when you have a window of time ready for you to take care of this issue. You'll want at least thirty minutes of quiet time to handle these cravings, ideally an hour at most. You will be handling some pretty substantial matters, so making sure that you're relaxed and able to come back to reality before and after the hypnosis will make it all the better.

The effectiveness varies from person to person. It will help you, and, on average, a person loses about six pounds. You might lose more, but you might not lose as much as expected. If you're trying to lose a ton of weight, this might not help. But, if you're looking to help eliminate cravings in your life and live a healthier lifestyle, then this is definitely the right tool for you. It's a way to help you supplement your exercising plans, and with this, you'll be able to have an even better time when it comes to shedding those pounds fast. There are other benefits of using hypnosis for weight loss. The obvious big one is that you lose weight. That's the one people will notice. You'll start to shed those pounds, and you might lose more than you expected. It won't be significant, such as like fifty pounds or more, but if you want to help your body and allow yourself the benefits of being able to control the cravings to lose weight, then this is perfect for you.

Then there are the lasting benefits of it. These are the benefits that you'll get because of the hypnosis. When you're doing this, you'll be able to tackle those parts of your subconscious that think it's okay to eat when you're stressed, or it'll tell you to eat more than necessary. Sometimes, your mind can be your own worst enemy, and this is undoubtedly one of those times. With hypnosis for weight loss, you'll allow yourself to handle your body in a positive manner. If you do this, you'll actually enable yourself to control your cravings and desires through the use of hypnosis. It might seem crazy, but it is possible. It's a great way to take life by the horns, and by doing this, you'll be able to allow yourself the benefit of controlling the factors in your life, such as stress or how much you eat, and turning them around to give yourself a more positive image that will benefit you in ways you've never expected before.

CHAPTER 1:

How Does the Mind Work?

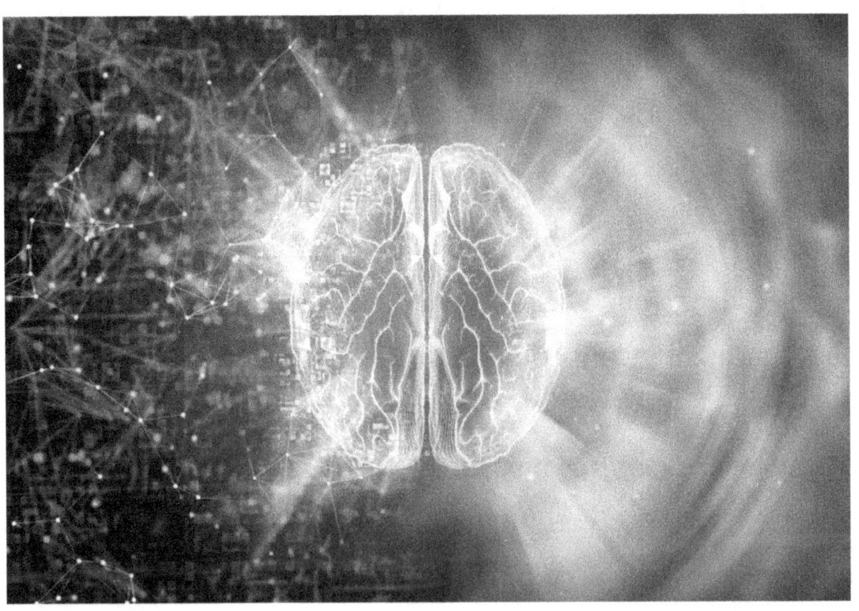

Perfect thoughts and ideal weight." The term may seem like a fantasy to you. Which is the ideal mind or ideal weight? They're the realistic conditions you'll be able to utilize as you pursue fat reduction. "Realistic?" You inquire. "How can anything be 'ideal,' let alone my burden and my ideas about my burden?" Well, recall what we said about the strength of believing and belief. Is it serving your curiosity to desire or hope for anything less than perfection on your own? Indulge us for some time as we clarify why you're able to think your mind and burden because "perfect."

Perfect fat is your weight that's ideal for you. It's the weight that's attainable and consistent with everything you need and precisely what you're ready to give yourself and accept yourself. More to the point, your ideal weight provides you with a healthy entire body, the human body which goes effortlessly, and also the one where you are feeling great about yourself and joyful. And what are ideal thoughts? You presently have a mind. It's flawless. But there can be a few ideas in that ideal thought of yours who are providing you with undesirable outcomes. There can be something that you keep in your mind, possibly habits or routines, which provide you with undesirable outcomes. However, you may use your ideal head to match your ideas to offer you precisely what you desire. It's possible to use your head to accomplish the bodyweight that you desire.

In the Twinkling of an Eye

Your current body is the consequence of your ideas and beliefs. You've behaved out these ideas and beliefs by your lifestyle, which generated your current weight. You haven't made any errors, regardless of what you may be thinking of yourself; instead, you've just experienced undesirable outcomes. These undesirable effects are an immediate effect of misaligned ideas and beliefs about yourself, which are very patterns of behavior or lifestyle. The Rapid Weight Loss Diet is all about utilizing your perfect thoughts

To align your ideas to provide you with the results you desire. You honestly can use your head to accomplish the bodyweight you desire. Let's examine a few of the learning which has occurred in your life, which has let you know where you're now together with your body weight. Do you wake up one afternoon, and you had been using the additional pounds? Or could it be a slow accumulation with time? Or perhaps you've understood nothing else as early youth. Whatever the situation, there are lots of factors that made your body:

- Food options

- Eating customs

- That the self-critic in you

- Economic history

- Psychological history

- Impact of household

- Impact of buddies

- Cultural heritage

These and several other variables were discovered in your life and eventually became the beliefs, which subsequently became routines of activity that generated your body. We'll be more specific. Notice that these aspects appear correct for you in your last years. In other words, consider what you did understand about your youth about eating and food.

What kinds of grocery stores did your household buy?

What foods did your kids cook, and were they typically ready?

Can you eat only at home or often grab food?

Have you been served fresh, healthy, high-calorie foods, or can you eat mainly processed and extremely processed foods, fried foods, and "junk" foods?

Was there an aware focus on nutrition, or has there been any irresponsible disregard for that which your household ate?

What did you find out about eating mindfully?

Were you educated that healthful food options led to healthy bodies?

Did anybody teach you how you can understand what's healthy food and what's not?

Are your meal selections based on which tasted or seemed high or priceless?

Can your loved ones or college instruct you about healthy lifestyles and audio nourishment, or has it been the "nutrition education" through TV advertisements and food makers' advertising?

What exactly did you learn as a kid? What're your beliefs about eating food, along with your entire body? Analyze your own socioeconomic or socio-cultural roots and see if they had an effect on the way and what you've learned to consume. Over thirty-five Years Back, sociological research pointed out weight issues in the working and lower class according to their intake patterns of what's been known as "poverty-level foods," like hot dogs, canned meats, and processed luncheon meats.

Cultural groups also have been analyzed to understand their nutritional patterns and meals, like eating with lard or ingesting a diet of fried and high-fat foods, which can lead to higher body fat loss. These influences can readily be accepted because they're "regular" into the category, of course. Then let's take a look at the teen years. During adolescence, are there some changes in your weight loss? Just as a boy, have you been invited to pile more food on your plate? "Look at him, consume! Certainly, he will develop to a large guy!" (There's a telling metaphor) Or are you currently admonished to eat? When you're a budding young woman, did a Smart girl take you under her wing and then with you that the marvel of menses and the wonderment of body modifications, such as the organic growth in body fat with all the evolution of breasts and broader hips?

Were you conscious during puberty, which unless the body improved body fat by 22 percent, it wouldn't correctly grow and create menses? Or was that "hushed up" within an awkward improvement? It was likely during adolescence which you heard there's a stigma involving obese individuals. Spend a couple of minutes writing down the aspects that appear to be accurate for you in your last years. Ponder the encounters and influences which are forming your body. In high school, the athletes at college sports have always been a healthful weight and are the cheerleaders and homecoming queens.

What ancient beliefs regarding your popularity and self-image could have formed from your social interactions in high school? What did you understand about physical activity, and what customs did you produce? Have you been introduced to physical activity as part of a healthy lifestyle, through family or sports outings of walks or hikes? Or was that the blaring TV a regular fixture, enticing everybody to the sofa? Next is a matter which most people have never been aware of throughout their development.

As you're growing up, has been that the attention of self-care based on trendy clothes, makeup, and hairstyles, or about healthful food, routine physical activity, along with spiritual and intellectual nourishment? What about today? Spend a couple more minutes writing down the aspects that appear to be accurate for you in the past couple of decades. What influences and experiences formed the ideas, which turned into the beliefs that turned into your body?

After high school, you moved away from the house. Suddenly you're no more captive to your family lifestyle. Can you be aware of your options, or can you start eating with blow off? If you input into a close connection, just what compromises or arrangements about foods and physical activity did you input into too? Most associations develop from similar pursuits, including food preferences and eating styles. In the end, the relationship comprises eating routines and tastes, which are a consequence of compromise.

Have your connections encouraged smart food choices and healthy eating? Maybe you've experienced pregnancy. Can you learn the way to get a wholesome pregnancy and then nourish a healthy infant within you? Or did you put in pounds? After giving birth, how did your lifestyle assist you in recovering your typical fat or suppressing it? If you were more active in the league or sports games, did your livelihood or family duties take priority and eliminate these physical fitness tasks from your regular? Can you correct exercise and diet so, or even did the fat begin to collect? Did an accident, injury, or disease happen that disrupted a standard physical action that has been supportive of healthy fat?

Because you can see, the way you got to where you're now was no crash. You heard from the folks about you--or you also consumed out of the surroundings --the best way to create food decisions, the way to eat, and the way to look after yourself emotionally and physically. Whether the thoughts you heard were tremendous and healthy or not so high and not as healthy, they became your own beliefs and eventually became you and the own human body because it is now. Bear in mind, and you didn't do something wrong; however, you need to experience the outcomes of eating and living, which have been consistent with your ideas and beliefs.

Through time, what's been your answer to individuals and their opinions about your weight loss, bad or good? Can you go out and purchase a fantastic pair of sneakers, or do you consume to facilitate psychological distress? Maybe you even heard the latter response in your youth.

Did your mom ever provide you with a plateful of food to comfort you when you're miserable? These are learned answers, and they may be unlearned and replaced with new answers and routines to make your ideal weight. Just ask, "Just how long does this happen?" We inform you, "In the twinkling of the eye," For the minute that you understand that you need it sufficient to get anything to possess it, it's completed. You've just altered the management of highly efficient energy in you and will redirect at figuring out how to attain the outcome which you need: your ideal weight.

Your Perfect Mind Relearning

It's simple to comprehend how you got or "heard" to contemplate over your ideal weight. And it'll be simple to create new decisions, to relearn new routines, and also to make new and much more healthful habits. How can we learn? We understand by mimicking another individual, analyzing books (such as that one) with different tools, and practicing the activities that create the outcomes we all seek. The best and lasting learning entails repetition and practice. The best way to practice is essential. Pretend for a minute that you're a violinist. You're searching for a grand symphony operation in New York.

Your piece includes five pubs, which are extremely difficult for your hands to perform appropriately. There are two ways that you practice. The first that is entirely ineffective would be to play with that steep fast, over and over and above, always playing precisely the very same mistakes, but trusting that your palms will play it properly. The next way to the clinic, which will always be active, would be to perform with the very, very slowly, mindfully "instruction" your hands the way to proceed, generating the "muscle " for the appropriate moves, before your palms have learned that the moves and may play with the whole segment correctly and in the appropriate pace with small if any, care focus. The critical point is that you're giving your focus on practicing correctly. By being aware of what you're practicing, and also the way you're practicing it, you're studying the new routines which are replacing the last routines.

Role of Human Mind in weight gain/loss

This chapter discusses in detail how a human brain can deceive you into gaining or losing weight. Triggers of overeating or underrating are discussed in this chapter. In order to attain optimal health, one should have a good relationship with food. Food should always be considered as a pleasant or joyful thing rather than giving it a name like food to reduce fat etc. This chapter will help you to overcome the negativity which you have for yourself so that you can live life to its fullest.

<u>The brain does make you fat</u>

Excess weight may feel like a thing of the belly, but your nervous system is among the major barriers to losing. What you feed, look and respond affects you whether or not you add weight. This is how the subconscious controls the body — and what you can do about it.

Anxiety fuels your needs.

Have a big presentation already come up, or are you about to have a challenging conversation with somebody you love? You should seek to control the discomfort; otherwise, you can catch yourself stopping the dinner otherwise preferred snack for a second. Sometimes referred to as stress feeding, fear causes this form of action and, when treated, may be counterproductive to the scale — both upward and downward.

Fear may have an overwhelming impact on the diet. Anxiety occurs differently in persons. Certain people will find themselves trying to regulate any ounce of food they consume, some may have the need to overeat, while some may lose their desire to eat completely.

Allowing negative to dominate

Within the head, the crystal-half-empty mentality may be challenging, but it often causes unhealthy habits of eating. Losing weight marketing is especially good for people who prey on the poor ways of thought that most people form about food.

The whole food industry is built to make consumers feel terrible for their health and make them believe they ought to waste all this money on a diet program that doesn't function.

Whenever the person's diet crashes, they feel bad for themselves and the process begins. People sometimes fault themselves for failing the diet, not the guy, when in fact it is. Before people get free of their eating habits, the body is hard to understand and everything that it offers, doesn't matter what big it might be.

Your brain turns dieting into fat preservation.

There are numerous misconceptions out there about weight reduction, but one aspect that is unequivocally real is that the brain avoids diet. Key brain cells actively prevent fat burning in the body when food is rare. A group of neurons in the brain coordinates appetite and energy spending and can turn on and off a switch to consuming or backup calories depending on what's in the environment available. We help us feed if food is abundant, and if food is unavailable, we transform our body into a survival mode to avoid from losing fat.

Depression triggers eating

Thinking processes causing obesity may be unconscious, but stress is an evident road to eating disorders. The weight gain is immutably related to the anxiety condition. Anxiety can significantly shift the culinary attitude and viewpoint. Depression feelings can manifest in excessive feeding or deprivation so what's important is resolving the head-on feelings. Recognizing what is going on is so crucial and finding professional treatment so that you really can take action not to allow stress to affect your well-being and weight.

Work destroys weight reduction targets

You can sense the cravings much more depressed than usual. And a brain under tension will indirectly weaken your attempts. If people feel uncomfortable regarding their bodies and eating patterns, the kinds of food they consume or the volume they consume can be unnecessarily limited. The body is created to live.

It doesn't realize why the human intentionally limits food, it only recognizes but it does not have sufficient, and it naturally slows down functions of the body, like metabolism, to save energy and to live. This physiological cycle often starts a primary urge to consume more to live, causing the individual to over-feed and struggle over food unconsciously.

Denying pleasure

Part of the weight-loss challenge is what products you choose to go there. If you're carelessly going for an apple because it's nice for you, however, it gives you a stomachache, why don't you make a move to eat a mango you'd like more?

Think about consuming an experience rather than a need. What that means is that by having the time to reflect on what you actually want to consume and make it a conscious activity, you allow yourself the chance to tune in and adapt to the nutritious meals that you would want to buy and enjoy, leaving you happy at mealtime.

Being judgmental

Will you feel a bad or a favorable connotation when you speak about a greasy burger and fries? How about a simple salad with hardly any treats? As we mature and start to assign various names to specific items, we start naming them accidentally — and sometimes, mindlessly —. Eliminating a 'good' behind such dishes and the 'evil' behind them will help shift the emphasis. "Food has little meaning, so feeding is not white and black. It has far less control over you, until the food has little moral obligation.

You don't even ask why

You remind yourself of something before you place the donut in your stomach. Is it food you desire — or anything else? "Enquire oneself if a meal is even whatever you need. People often crave comfort and support when eating without body hunger. It's fine to eat at a family party for selfish reasons, like cake, but you have to be capable to identify those signs and make a decision for yourself whether food is that you need or want or whether anything else will assist you accordingly.

Just to tap into gratitude

Humility can boost your well-being in several respects, but it's difficult to be thankful to oneself. Whenever an eating spree begins a cycle of shame, look at how incredible it is our brain and heart function to keep us healthy instead of throwing themselves a hard time. It gives sense why, if we build shortages by dieting, certain biological forces be in high gear to save our resources and lead us to search for high-calorie foods — or normally foods that we've resisted. What if we all quit dieting nonsense and chose to take control of our body and function through our appetite rather than battle it? Instead, in a range of body types and ages, we will find much healthier individuals who kept fairly healthy weights and enjoyed improved fitness.

Confidence won't support you

If you really can't turn your mind the correct way around? And do not be scared to ask somebody who is able to tackle something that delays your development, for assistance. Trying to break the dietary and food anxiety mental loop is challenging, it requires training and experience. A nutritionist who specializes in mindful eating as well as the — anti-diet method will assist you on the journey.

How to lose weight using your mind?

If you've ever attempted weight reduction, you realize that consuming nutritious food and exercising your body are essential elements of every weight-loss strategy. Yet have you learned that reaching or sustaining a balanced body structure exists both in the body and mind? In fact, if you've repeatedly tried to lose some weight but never succeeded or you lose the weight and then regain the weight (and then some!), your thoughts and beliefs — not your diet — are most likely holding you back. This is because the extra weight is a result of the state of mind or sentiment. And the main reason people struggle to lose weight is that they ignore to implement adjustments in their subconscious mind in order to support their conscious objectives.

How to Reshape Your Figure with Your Thoughts

Listen to your self-talk.

Self-respect and recognition of oneself are the key elements for reaching optimum weight. Yet, most individuals cannot lose weight when participating in body-shaming talk and actions.

It's crucial to learn if you spoke about yourself before attempting to lose weight. Whether you tell your body you dislike how it appears for much of your life or scratch your face in the mirror in frustration that someone used to do that to you, the subconscious mind would accept the emotional conditioning. You will reconfigure your subconscious mind by communicating with your body in a constructive, caring manner — the way you'd be communicating to an innocent kid.

Look in the mirror to see what the body likes. Touch the parts you want to change, and say, "Thank you for keeping me alive."

Make sure your body loses weight safely. Perform so every single day. Through time, the subconscious can comply with the urge to shed weight, actively.

Say affirmations.

Affirmations tend to reinforce your trust in the latest tale; you are designing the subconscious. When they are convincing, they do work well. Yet if you think, "I'm going to be 80 pounds thinner in a month," your amygdala won't accept it. Instead, try to say, "I become the super fit person that lives inside me! "And claim, 'I'm making good choices now that reflect my ideal weight.' You might also create a routine of voicing your comments. For example, you can smudge stagnant energy in your room or home, light candles, sit with your closed eyes, and say your statements three times in a row. Practice these two to three times a day. You may want to repeat another variation of your comments right before you feel sleepy when your subconscious mind is more open to advice. Remember, the affirmations have to be as if they had already manifested in the present tense. Affirmations will not trigger something to happen. They accept everything.

Try Tapping.

The Emotional Freedom Technique (EFT) or Tapping, helps match the subconscious mind with the expectations on an optimistic basis by resolving the unconscious feelings, habits, values, traumas, and more than that contribute to weight gain. You begin by stating your current restricting conviction preceded by expressing how you enjoy and support yourself while taping on different points of acupressure. For starters, you might claim, "I love and truly support myself even if I have a difficult time trying to lose weight." This removes stress levels in the body and can remove the negative emotions and values connected with the extra pounds, and you can break old patterns and recover.

Identify Your 'Trouble Thoughts'

Identify the thoughts that cause you trouble and fight to eliminate and alter it. Maybe if you look into a mirror, it's your inner voice. Or cravings when stressed out. Let them avoid knowingly by saying 'no' out loud. It may sound silly, but that simple action breaks your chain of thought and allows you to introduce something new or healthier. The best approach to do this is to count as many as you need from one to 100 times until the damaging thoughts fade.

Eat mindfully.

Research suggests that stress reduction — concentrated knowledge of your emotions, behaviors, and intentions — plays an important role in weight reduction in the long term when combined alongside certain weight loss approaches. Learn alertness when you cook and enjoy your food.

Seek to be aware of starvation and plenitude thoughts. Pay close attention to flavors, textures, and the munching as well as gulping actions of your food. Be conscious also of how the body sounds after consuming those foods.

This exercise will help lower binge and raise an understanding of behaviors that do not benefit the weight-loss goals. So, if you try to connect what you eat to how you feel, you're not going to have to eat normally to lose weight. It is going to happen mercilessly.

Also, your body composition and body image will be transformed when you learn from your mistakes about food as body-nourishment. When you link with your body and nurture it from an area of empathy and self-respect, the emotions focused on self-respect create in your body a metabolic environment conducive to ideal fat burning.

Address Yourself Like You Would a Friend

We are extremely tough on ourselves whenever it comes to beauty ideals and body image.

The expectations we set for ourselves are harsh. So, we should never have kept many of those requirements to our peers or loved ones. You receive the same consideration so kindness as everyone else; handle yourself like that.

Throw Out the Calendar

Patience is also important when you lose weight in a healthy and sustainable matter. Plus, if you focus on achieving genuinely actionable goals, such as taking 10,000 steps each day, and no need to get tangled up in a timeline of goals ahead.

Say "good-bye" to Energy Vampires.

One of the most striking things that have been observed in the relationships among both vampires and sensitive people is the discrepancy in their tendencies to gain weight. Your life and relationships represent your capacity to nurture yourself. If you are in a variant relationship where you constantly give and try to please some other individual, your efforts to lose weight will become in vain because you are using the energy of your vampire (which can be a state—not a person). This causes even more stress and cortisol and takes your own energy. As a result, you look out for sugar, carbs, and/or alcohol. And you will keep on gaining weight no matter what you do—even when you eliminate the carbohydrates because the weight acts as an extra layer of "self-protection.

Take a Breath

Taking a few minutes of stability at the beginning of your workout, or even at the beginning of your day, slowing down and simply focusing on the act of breathing can help you create your intentions, link with your body, and even lower the response to the stress of your body. Lie down with legs stretched and place one hand on your stomach and one on your chest. Inhale for four seconds, hold for two and then exhale through the mouth for six seconds. With each breath, the hand kept on your stomach should be the only one to rise or fall.

Designed to Eat

So why is it really so hard to reduce weight? The human body and brain are meant to eat explaining why weight loss proves so difficult for so many people. The factors of obesity are complicated. Obesity is not merely a laziness trait or an indicator of mental dysfunction. Therefore, hereditary and biological influences do not function in isolation but work with a variety of environmental variables on a permanent basis. Both the accessibility and persuasive advertising of unsafe food contribute to the epidemic of obesity.

CHAPTER 2:

The secret to lasting weight loss

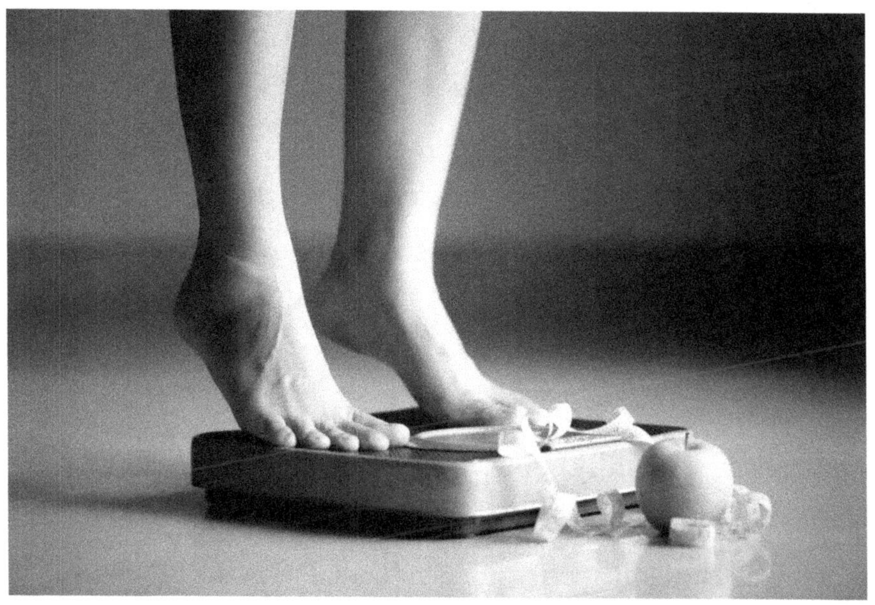

This script will help you maintain your weight loss. Weight maintenance is one of the hardest parts of weight loss, so many people can lose weight but struggle to keep the changes that they've made because of the challenges that naturally come when people have lost the weight and think, "Oh, the diet is over."

While you can make some dietary changes when you've lost weight and be less strict with yourself, you can never return to the bad habits that made you gain weight in the first place. Thus, hypnosis can give your unconscious brain the suggestions it needs to keep your weight steady once you have lost it.

Starter Script

You can stay healthy. Believe that you have the will to keep going. Sometimes, it gets hard, but you are resilient. You have created all the skills that you need to deal with the burdens that will try to drag you down. You are going to get through any hardship that comes your way because you believe in yourself, and you know how powerful your mind is. Your mind will guide you automatically when you are tired or are feeling defeated.

Now that you have taught it the skills it needs; it will try to further those skills even when you're at your most vulnerable. Repeat this message when you feel yourself slipping, "I am strong, and I can handle whatever life throws at me without returning to my old ways."

Give yourself breaks when you mess up. Do your best but be reasonable with yourself. Let yourself be human. You will not push yourself to do anything that will hurt you in the long run, even in the name of maintaining your weight. If you overeat, you will not turn to methods like purging or restriction.

You will continue to give your body what it needs, and you will not punish it. Instead of trying to make up for your slip-ups, you will choose to do better next time rather than torturing yourself over accidents because you'll always make mistakes no matter how long after you have lost the weight.

These messages will become part of you. You will listen to the notions that I have given because they will make you stronger. Let them settle into your brain and create new paths in your mind that will help you be successful at weight maintenance. Emerge from your trance and let yourself accept the suggestions that you have taken into your mind during this process.

Intermediate Script

Listen closely to the messages that I will give. These suggestions will encourage you to keep up the diligent work. Relax and let your thoughts calm. They will still make noise but focus on what you can do to improve your mind rather than silence it altogether. Let yourself be engaged in this process and find a new way of thinking.

When you have temptation, you will not give in. Think about all the things you can earn when you don't let temptation control you. Keep in mind the things you would lose if you gave up and let yourself go back to how you were. You don't want to go backward.

You want to continue forward using the momentum that you got from your weight loss. Let yourself improve and find victory beyond just weight loss. If you gain weight again, you'll have to start at square one, and that can be one of the least motivating places to be.

You've made it so far. There's no reason to go back. Don't be one of the people who fail to keep lost weight off. Choose to be one of the successful ones because failing will never make you feel good about yourself. If you can keep the weight off, you will prove to yourself that you are empowered to channel your mental energy into doing more extraordinary things.

If you gain the weight back, you will doubt your abilities and will stagnate yourself based on those doubts. Whatever weight you are doesn't matter, but it's the way you feel based on that weight that needs to change first and foremost. Funnily enough, having confidence that you lose and keep off weight is the thing you need to lose and keep off weight. You will keep it off if you remind yourself you will.

Remember all the people who are supporting you. Show them that you can succeed. Don't disappoint yourself and the people who helped you by self-sabotaging and returning to your old weight. You deserve permanent change for yourself more than others, but you still need to appreciate the help you got along the way.

Remind yourself of why you want to keep going and push yourself to maintain all the good habits you have created. Never quit bettering yourself. You have so much potential to unlock and embracing that potential and continuing to improve will help you resist reverting to your old self.

You're doing so well, so continue to do by embracing these suggestions. They will benefit you for years going forward and make it easier to maintain the good habits that you have created during your weight loss journey. Snap out of your trance and continue your day with the messages I have given to you.

Advanced Script

Use the suggestion in this script to reaffirm your goal to lose and keep the weight off. Take a big breath through your nose and close your eyes. Let yourself feel the inner stillness that allows you to focus on vital subconscious thoughts that you want to target. Breathe into a peaceful state, and let your mind emphasize these important messages that I will present to you right now.

You are so close to being where you've been working to be, so keep going. Continue bettering your brain in ways that have the most significant impact. When you boost your mind, you also nurture your body, so don't neglect your brain now that your body has changed.

You will get your beauty sleep. You will continue to get seven to eight hours of sleep per night because it is easier to keep up all the other good habits when you are well-rested. Your rest is not something that you will sacrifice. You will value it as a refreshing time for your body. Sleep is not an option. If you want to keep the weight off, you need it. Give yourself breaks, both mental and physical to keep in top shape.

Think of yourself in bed and imagine the calm you would feel as you sleep. Visualize your body, reinforcing itself for the next day. It is assembling an invisible armor around you that will protect you from your vulnerabilities and all the things that you can't foresee. Sleep builds that armor, and without it, you are prone to attacks. You'll feel more emotionally hungry if you don't sleep, so let yourself sleep even if you have a million things to do.

You will eat healthily. You cannot stop eating well just because you have lost weight. You will continue to make smart decisions about your diet. You will have foods that have nutrients and keep your body balanced. You will let yourself have treats, but you will not let those treats overrun your life and become coping mechanisms.

Visualize all the delicious meals that you will have. Imagine a table with heaps of colorful food. You can choose whatever foods you want. You can have a little bit of each food if you desire, but you can't eat it all without hurting yourself. If you eat it all, your stomach will grow, and you'll feel uncomfortably full and bloated. However, if you only choose what you need and a little of what you desire, you will feel great. You will have energy and peace of mind. You won't have to feel guilty when you do indulge.

You will continue to exercise. You'll let activities that make you happy continue to be a part of your life. You will enjoy the liberation you feel like your body moves and changes because of your workouts. Imagine your body moving smoothly and freely. Think of yourself as a feather gliding through the wind. You are not inhibited by anything weighing you down. You can push against the wind and steer where you are going.

Exercise gives you that lightness because it allows your body to do more incredible things. You will do greater things. You will push your body to do more things than you thought it could do. Your body is precious, so you won't force it to work out to the point of insanity, but you will let it have the rush of endorphins that come with being active.

You will keep the weight off. The excess weight will never be back on your body because you won't let it be. You will shove away all the things that threaten to bring the weight back. You will push through your fears and doubts to remain the weight you are happiest and healthiest at.

Think of how good you will feel when you have freedom from your weight. You'll feel calmer and more confident than ever when you have learned to love your body in all its sizes, but mainly its healthiest size.

Weight loss shouldn't be a fix-all. It won't cure your problems, but it can give you the state of mind you need to transform yourself from the inside out. Maintain your weight because weight loss is a tool you used to propel yourself forward in life. You will never be the size you hated again because you will do what it takes to maintain your weight loss.

You will let these suggestions into your subconscious. Permit them to take a permanent space in your head and serve as important reminders. They will solidify the progress you have made, and they will ensure that you lose weight for life. Your journey is not over. It never is, but you have made substantial progress, and you only must deal with the easy part of weight loss now— living your life and finding a new normal. Curate better habits and continue to force yourself to grow.

You will not let yourself stagnate. You will discover pursuits beyond weight loss. Weight loss will be just another part of your past, and weight maintenance will be a small but essential part of your daily life. You are more formidable and fitter than ever. Go out into the world and let yourself be happy, healthy, and feel less heavy. Emerge from your trance, and go live the good life!

Healthy Habits Are a Must

The habits you have make a difference in your weight loss, and these are many of the area's hypnosis will help you tackle, but you also need to be aware of the influence of these areas before you even begin hypnosis. The better handle you have on these parts of your life going into hypnosis, the more effectively your hypnosis will work. You need to have clear goals of what you expect of yourself. Determine how you want to handle each area better to promote the most success based on your personal experiences and needs.

Diet

Diet is probably the most essential addition to your hypnosis. All the research that has been done on hypnosis and weight loss has shown you need to have a good diet plan to do well with weight loss through hypnosis. The diet plan you choose is up to you, but there are many mistakes people make when trying to establish a diet. Often, they create unrealistic expectations for themselves, which inevitably leads to failure on their part. Be honest with yourself when you are planning your diet. Know what you'll be able to stick to, and know what parameters would drive you too crazy to handle in the long-term.

Keep a balanced diet. You need to have balance no matter what diet you choose, which means you need to maintain a variety of foods in your diet plan. Sure, eating a calorie-restricted diet plan of only candy will, in theory, lead to weight loss, but that diet plan would not be conducive to long-term change. You would become deficient in a variety of vitamins and minerals, and your body would practically beg you to eat other foods.

You'd end up eventually breaking your diet and returning to your old habits. The pounds would all go back on, and all that time you spent eating just one candy would be wasted. If you have the nutrients that you need, you are less likely to have those intense cravings that derail you from progress and make you feel like a failure.

Don't over restrict your food. When you become limiting with your diet, that's when it becomes hard to stick to it. There's no need to cut out your favorite foods. If you love potato chips, you don't need to cut them out altogether. Try to eat less of them, but you don't need to say, "I will never eat a potato chip again," because that is unrealistic. You aren't going to be able to resist them for the rest of your life.

Make changes that allow flexibility and that you can continue long past when you've lost all the weight you want to lose. It would help if you were trying to make lifestyle changes, not temporary ones. Successful diets don't have an end date. They continue for the rest of your life. That may sound grim, but once you change your habits, it won't feel so awful, especially if you make livable changes.

Carbs are not evil. For whatever reason, diet culture has furthered the idea carbs are bad for you. Yes, simple cards like sweets and white bread are not as nutritionally dense as other foods, but whole grains should be a vital part of your diet, and you should allow yourself to have simple carbs occasionally too.

Your body needs carbs to function because carbs are what fuel your brain. When you don't eat carbs, you may feel worse, and you will probably crave them because your body instinctually knows what it needs. Thus, instead of trying to cut carbs out, try to eat more complex carbohydrates like brown rice, wheat bread, or whole wheat pasta.

Fat isn't evil either. Since the 1980s, the diet industry has demonized fat, maybe even worse than carbs. Again, this rhetoric is inaccurate. While trans fats and saturated fats should be limited, your body does need fat. Fat is what your body uses to energize you between meals when you have burned through your carbs.

Fat also pads your organs and protects them. When you don't have enough fat, your body will begin eating muscles, including your heart! Low-fat diets can harm your body. Aim to include polyunsaturated fats and monounsaturated fats into your diet.

Proteins are also vital. These keep your muscles healthy, and they also have a myriad of diverse functions around your body. Aim to eat lean proteins like chicken or lean fish. Alternatively, you can eat plant-based proteins like soybeans (or tofu) or combine starch and legume/ seed to make a full protein (i.e. rice and beans). You'll want to eat proteins several times throughout the day because protein cannot be stored in your body, which is why trends like intermittent fasting can leave you feeling worse than if you were to have smaller meals throughout the day.

Don't forget your micronutrients! Vitamins and minerals are essential to your health because they keep your bodily functions such as vision and digestive health going. They also make sure you can use your muscles and that your heart can beat properly. They are part of all your systems, and you can be sure to get them through fruits and vegetables. Try to eat produce that is of a variety of colors and types to ensure that you get all the vitamins and minerals you need for your body to work as it should.

When you have a healthy diet, you will feel better all-around in your life. Plus, you will be taking the steps that you need to further your weight loss. Strive for satiety rather than trying to cut several foods out of your diet. You don't need to eat only vegetables and protein to be healthy. You can eat everything, but you merely have to change the way you eat those things. Incorporate more "good" things rather than eliminating all the "bad." Stop villainizing food. There aren't good or bad foods. You can have them all. Some foods are more nutritious than others while you should eat others in moderation.

Exercise

Exercise is another excellent way to promote a healthy lifestyle that you need for weight loss. Physical activity is a great mood booster that can help you feel better in your skin. It also allows you to replace fat with muscle so that you can tone your body.

When you exercise, you combine the powers of your mind with the capabilities of your body, and you build yourself up. Exercise is not just about your body, which is something that people don't always realize. Some physical activity allows you to be in a better headspace and to feel all-around better about yourself and your condition. The health benefits of exercise are extensive. By just adding a little bit of exercise a day, you can better your cardiovascular health. Even just an additional fifteen-minute walk can make you less likely to have heart disease. Further, it reduces your blood pressure, which makes you more resistant to stress. Some studies indicate that active people can reduce their risk of conditions like diabetes and cancer. Plus, being regularly active increases your immune function, making you less prone to illness in general. When you are more active, you'll probably feel better even if you can't see the changes in your body right away. People who exercise often get better quality sleep and can sleep longer, which is incredibly important to your health. You also feel mentally better when you exercise and are less depressed and anxious because of the feel-good endorphins that exercise sends through your body. Best of all, people who exercise live longer. You can't go wrong with exercise!

You don't need to start crazy workouts to be healthy. Find ways to enjoy exercise. You don't have to be a star athlete to reap the benefits of exercise. Anyone can improve their lives by just adding a little more activity. It doesn't have to be an organized workout either. Dancing in your living room or going for a bike ride through a park also counts even though they don't feel as scary as more intense activities. Do what makes you feel good and you'll be able to stick to it. You can build up to more workouts later if you are so inclined. When you live a more active life, you become happier and healthier. You also can lose weight when you add in more activity. Exercise can improve your life experiences in so many ways you won't realize until you add it consistently to your life.

Sleep

Sleep is one of the most critical parts of your overall health. People who get more sleep have better health outcomes, both physical and mental. The impacts of sleep on your health carry many of the same benefits of exercise. People who get more sleep tend to live longer. They also have better heart health. When you sleep, you feel less stressed and can deal with anxiety better. You feel ready to take on the world rather than wanting to ignore all your issues.

You are less moody when you sleep, so it is easier to keep your spirits up and avoid the pull of emotional eating. If you make no other change in this eBook, change your sleep because when you aren't sleeping, your body struggles to function. Driving when you are sleep deprived can be as bad as driving drunk, which shows how dangerous not getting sleep is!

Additionally, you tend to reach for foods that take less energy to prepare, which usually means junk food that does not fill you because it is nutritionally empty. Alternatively, leptin is the hormone that makes you feel full. When your body sends leptin through your body, you know you've had enough food; however, when you are tired, your body doesn't produce as much leptin.

Thus, with the rush of ghrelin and little leptin, you are hungrier and don't feel as satiated regardless of the amount of food that you are eating. Further, when you are tired, you are more emotional, so you might eat food to deal with feelings because you are too exhausted to cope with them in any other way. You'll want the nutritionally empty foods you habitually choose. As a result, getting sleep is a crucial part of managing your body's hunger cues and cravings.

Do not underestimate the value of sleep. Sleep is something that people often try to skip. They think that they are too busy to take eight hours from their schedule for sleep. If you want hypnosis to work and to lose weight, you need to take care of your body and get your rest in. If you don't, you will not be in the headspace to respond well to treatment.

Your body will fight against you even more than it would normally. You have time to sleep. Watch less TV, and you'll probably quickly find a little more time to sleep. We're all busy, but when we get to sleep, we can be more productive during the hours that we do work. Tired people take forever to get anything done.

Mental Health

To make lasting changes, you need to address your mental health. Hypnosis can help you improve your mental health, but it targets specific areas, so if you have issues beyond your weight that you need to address, find ways to manage them. Don't let your emotional wounds keep hurting you. It is time to move on and get better.

Share your past hurts with a friend, loved one, or a therapist. Don't run away from your problems. It would be best if you faced the things that hurt you and owned up to the things that fuel your inability to lose weight. Be kinder to yourself. Stop beating yourself

CHAPTER 3:

How to use meditation to beat food cravings

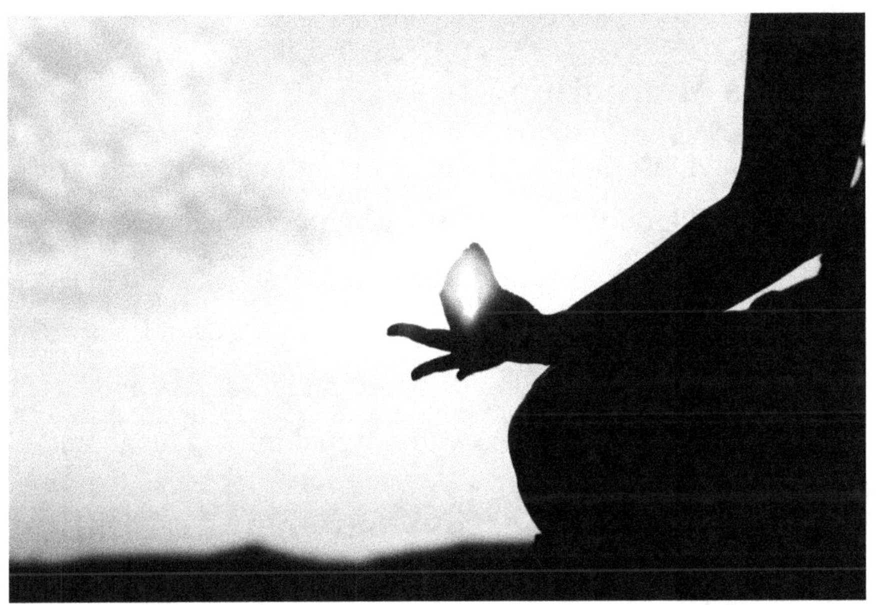

When it comes to rapid weight loss, meditation is one of the techniques that act like secret weapons. Studies conducted on meditation and mindfulness have shown that these exercises are linked to weight loss. They not only boost an individual's awareness but also banish belly fat and lower stress levels. Having an attentive mind can help you avoid binge or emotional eating.

What is Meditation?

Meditation must not be a difficult technique. If you are a beginner, take only five minutes when you wake up to clear your mind before you start off your day. You just need to close your eyes and focus your mind on your goals as you breathe in and out. As you breathe, don't let your mind wander, and if this happens simply guide it back without making any judgment.

What is the Connection between Meditation and Weight Loss?

Meditation is known to be an effective tool for weight loss. It aligns the unconscious mind with the conscious mind in order to facilitate changes that we want to make in our behaviors. Such changes may include avoiding unhealthy foods by altering them with healthier foods. It is important that your unconscious mind becomes engaged in the change process because it is where the weight-gaining, poor habits such as emotional eating are cultivated. Through meditation, you will be able to become more aware of your surroundings and will be able to overcome your unhealthy habits.

But there is even a more immediate effect of mediation. It can reduce the level of stress hormones in the body. Hormones like cortisol give the body signal to store more calories. If you have high levels of cortisol moving through your system, it is going to be difficult to cut down weight even if you are eating healthy foods. Most of us are stressed in most cases, but it takes only 25 minutes of meditation three times in arrow to reduce the effects of stress.

In 2016, a study that was conducted by Texas Tech University found that increased relaxation, attention, body-mind awareness, calmness, and brain activity result from just a few sessions of meditation. The study also suggested that your self-control could increase with daily meditation. The researchers found that the brain is most affected by meditation, which means that with a few minutes of meditation, you will be able to pass by that ice cream when feeling stressed.

How to Start Meditating for Weight Loss

Even without training, anyone who has a body and mind can practice meditation. For most of us, the most challenging aspect of meditation is getting time. You can start with as little as 8 to 10 minutes a day.

Ensure that you are able to access a quiet place for meditation. If you have children or other people around you, you may need to squeeze time when they are not awake or after they have left the house to avoid distractions. You may even practice your mediation while in the shower.

Once you are in a place of silence, take a comfortable position. You can either lie down or sit in a position that makes you feel at ease.

Start meditating by putting your focus on your breath. Watch the way your stomach or chest rises and falls. Feel the air that you breathe in and out of your mouth. Listen keenly to the sounds around you. This should be done for 2 or 3 minutes until you begin feeling relaxed.

Next, do the following steps:

- Take in a deep breath, and hold for a few seconds

- Slowly breathe out, and repeat the process

- Breathe in a natural manner

- Observe the way your breath enters your nostrils, influence the movement of your chest, and moves your stomach.

- Continue focusing on the way you breathe in and out for about 8 to 10 minutes

- Your mind may begin to wonder, which a normal occurrence is. Just acknowledge this and return your attention back to the process

- As you wrap up, reflect on your thoughts, and acknowledge how you can easily bring your mind together

Benefits of Meditation on Weight Loss

Below are the incredible ways that meditation can help you achieve daily weight loss:

<u>Meditation reduces stress</u>

With meditation, you will feel calmer as well as have a stress-reducing impact on your body. With endless roles in life including work, children, and home activities, it is not surprising that you may be overwhelmed, which may contribute to increased stress. Unfortunately, these stressors affect your body by producing more cortisol, a stress hormone that affects the levels of sugar and insulin in the body. As a result, the hormone causes weight gain. Studies have revealed that meditation activates a relaxation response, regulating the nervous system and, in turn, lowering the cortisol levels.

With a few minutes of deep breathing and conscious relaxation, you will be able to obtain the cortisol-lowering benefits as well as your overall stress levels.

Meditation promotes a focus on intention

Often, meditation techniques involve focusing on specific goals or concepts. Meditating on cutting down weight streams your energy, thoughts, and intentions to a particular goal. In this case, you submit to the intentions by revealing your goals to the world, which makes both your conscious and subconscious mind to be aware of the goal that you want to lose some weight. The outspoken intention will stay with you for a long while, enabling you to achieve your weight loss goal both consciously and subconsciously, and dodging all possible distractions.

With meditation, you will learn conscious eating

With daily meditation, you will be able to boost your levels of mindfulness and awareness. This can allow you to live in the moment and always focus on what you are doing in the present. The process of meditation can help you gain an increased sense of awareness of actions and thoughts, thus helping you to think twice before you have taken action. Rather than enabling your cravings to take over you, you will develop the power of controlling your mind, thus handling your cravings with greater intention and awareness. When you are ready to eat, your awareness will make it easier to recognize the textures and flavors of the food you are eating, instead of taking them for granted.

Meditation stabilizes mood hormones

Common daily stressors and activities can affect the way your system operates normally and may throw your hormones out of normal functioning. Apart from keeping your cortisol and adrenaline levels regulated, meditation goes further than this. The technique for relaxation releases both oxytocin and serotonin hormones, which boost your moods and ensure your hormones remain stable.

Meditation regulates sleep

Lack of sleep may hinder your weight loss progress. You see, by having a deep sleep, your cortisol levels will rise, which in turn will sabotage your progress in losing weight. Also, when you lack sleep, ghrelin, a hunger signal hormone, is also produced in plenty, thereby increasing your chances of eating more for weight gain. With meditation, you will be able to balance the circadian rhythms that promote quality sleep. Meditation increases the levels of melatonin, a hormone that also determines and controls when you sleep.

How to Make Sure that Meditation Works for You

If you want to include meditation in your rapid weight loss hypnosis, it is important that you make it simple. Meditation should help you recover from any stressful event, not become a source of it. That is why you need to consider the three easy ways highlighted below, which you can incorporate in your daily mediation.

Consider a Mantra That Can Help You Lose Weight

A mantra refers to a phrase that one repeats to focus their mind on mediation and bring them to a relaxation state. A mantra can give help you identify something to focus on as you meditate. Although it is very helpful to many people, a mantra is not a must in meditation. You don't need to force yourself to use one if you don't find it helpful or if it does not make you feel natural. However, in case you choose to use one, you need to repeat it as you inhale as well as when you exhale. Some of the common mantras used include "I am at peace with myself," "I am loved," or "I can do this."

Follow Your Breath to Avoid Stress

As you meditate, try to count your inhales 4 times and exhales 8 times. Remember that meditation is a process that is aimed at reducing stress; if these counts do not feel natural, you should deviate from them. Every time you meditate, always try to increase the number of exhaling and inhaling counts. Do not feel stressed if it takes longer to reach 8 counts. Just keep in mind that lengthening the exhale will greatly affect your health as you will be able to calm down.

Consider a Guided Meditation

If you are not able to practice meditation alone, you should consider a guided process. This includes websites, phone apps, podcasts, and recordings that can help you connect with experts who guide you on how to meditate.

How to Create a Meditation Space at Home

You may find it easier to practice meditation on a daily basis to motivate your weight loss process. Creating and incorporating meditation accessories and organizing the right space might help you throughout the practice. Some of the equipment to get started including:

Essential Oil Diffuser

Aromatherapy is considered an effective calming tool for the body, which is very helpful during meditation. An essential oil diffuser can help you create a relaxing environment in order to reap the benefits of the essential oils. Additionally, the diffuser always shuts off when the water runs out; thus, you can meditate as long as you like.

Bluetooth Earbud Headphones

Don't have enough space to practice your meditation? You may consider wireless headphones, which you can to wherever you go.

The headphones can sync up with Android and iPhones devices, which you can use to listen to your best-guided mediation without bothering those close to you.

A Meditation Filled Cotton Pillow Cushion

A meditation cushion can give you the comfort to find a point of relaxation. The cushion will relieve you from stress, especially after having a prolonged sitting period. It has the perfect density and height to sit through for hours of meditation practice.

Meditation That Will Burn Your Fats

Our bodies were designed to burn fat. It is the way that they provide the body with energy when we haven't given it enough through the foods we eat. We require more energy when we workout, so our bodies will burn more fat during these processes.

Though it can sound so simple on paper, it will be rather challenging to always include these things in our lives.

This meditation is going to help guide you through the journey of getting the body you want, with a visualization exercise to help you see your goals laid out clearly. Listen to this first when you are in a relaxed position in case you become calm to the point of sleep.

After you know how you react, you might include this when you are doing yoga or another form of light exercise to help keep you grounded and relaxed.

Meditation and Daily Habits

People become emotionally attached to food from infancy through adulthood. Children sometimes get rewarded with snacks or treats for healthy behavior; adults can be treated to dinner. There are so many celebrations across the year from Christmas, Halloween, Thanksgiving, birthdays, and Valentine's Day. All these celebrations are food-focused, and as people eat together, they feel good and happy.

It has also been proven that an aroma of a special kind of baked cake can create an emotional connection memory that will last throughout someone's lifetime. Some foods are for nourishment, but others we take just for comfort, depending on how they make us feel. Whenever the brain reacts and feels pleasure for a particular food within our reach, most of the time, we will grab it and eat it. During this time, the brain releases a chemical called dopamine, the process feels perfect, and if we equate the feeling with food, then the outcome will be negative.

High body mass index (BMI) can be linked to emotional problems like anxiety, depression, and stress. Those emotional issues can make one overindulge after a rough day at the office as a reward for a good feeling. Some people use junk food as a coping mechanism when they hear bad news. This habit can be only be improved by the use of meditation exercises to deal with one's emotions, stress, or anxiety. As the practices continue and you pay close attention to your breath and allocate more time for thinking.

Tackling Barriers to Weight Loss

There are so many barriers to weight loss from personal, to medical, to support system and emotional health. Meditation, if incorporated, will bring fruitful and healthy results. Dedication to overcome the challenges and to be focused on achieving your goals is significant. There are so many distractions, especially before you start tour weight loss routine.

It takes discipline and resilience to manage a healthy loss program. We need to give weight loss the priority it deserves. Also, we need to realize the existence of the said barriers and their contribution toward our goal. The barriers will determine our successes and failures.

Set realistic goals

When you set goals, ensure that they are attainable, specific, and realistic. It is effortless to work on realistic goals and achieve them for better results. If the goals are unrealistic; however, the success rate will be low since one will be discouraged. For instance, when starting with meditation, you can start with as little as five minutes a day and gradually increase it daily until you reach the maximum time like sixty minutes.

The same applies to lose weight during the meditation process. You can start focusing on losing a few pounds each week and gradually increase until you reach your goal. As you set goals, however, realize that it is not your fault if they do not work out as you had planned, do your best and keep your focus.

Always be Accountable

Once you have decided to commit to meditation for weight loss, don't shy away from sharing your plan with your support system and family. It is to ensure that the people you share with also reinforce the commitment and form part of the support system. That way, they will feel part of the program and give support whenever there is a need. You can also use apps for reminders and timings; this way, you have a backup plan whenever you forget.

You can also use motivational bands whenever you achieve a milestone set. Being accountable makes you enjoy your successes, acknowledge your failure, and appreciate your support system.

People thrive when they feel responsible for something, especially for something beneficial to their well-being.

Modify Your Mindset

Your thinking needs to be modified in the sense that you be keen on the information you are telling yourself. Ensure that your mind is not filled with unproductive and negative thoughts, which will bring you down or discourage you. Do not be scared of challenging your thoughts and appreciate your body image.

Your mindset determines your thinking and in turn, creates a sense of appreciation or rejection. Our weight loss largely depends on our mindset; do you believe you can do it? If you think you have all it takes, then absolutely nothing will prevent or stop you.

Manage Stress Regularly

Having a stress management technique should be part of one's daily routine. You need to develop a healthy stress-relieving mechanism that can help you live a stress-free life. Understand that meditation is a stress reliever in its own right as it helps calm the mind and soothes the body.

It can be used to manage stress and its benefits fully utilized to live a more productive life. Be able to handle stress efficiently. Stress is not healthy for the mind.

If not handle, it can cause emotional problems and makes one irrational, moody, or violent. Be your own boss when managing your stress.

Be Educated About Weight Loss

As you embark on meditation for weight loss, be educated about how it works; that way, weight loss will not be a struggle.

You will be able to handle failed attempts as well as appreciate the progress made.

You will be able to know what you have been doing wrong and decide on the best meditation exercise for you.

If you have misleading information, then your general progress may be inhibited

Weight loss need not be too expensive; neither does it require a costly gym membership or enrolment in a costly meditation class. There are various self-practice meditation exercises that you can comfortably do at home. There are various meal plans and diets that may work for others though they may not offer long-term solutions or lasting behavior changes. Have the right information that you need. Don't be misled by anyone posing that they are professionals in that field. Also, do not hesitate to do research online and compare notes. From there, you will be able to come back with something that works for you.

CHAPTER 4:

What is Hypnosis?

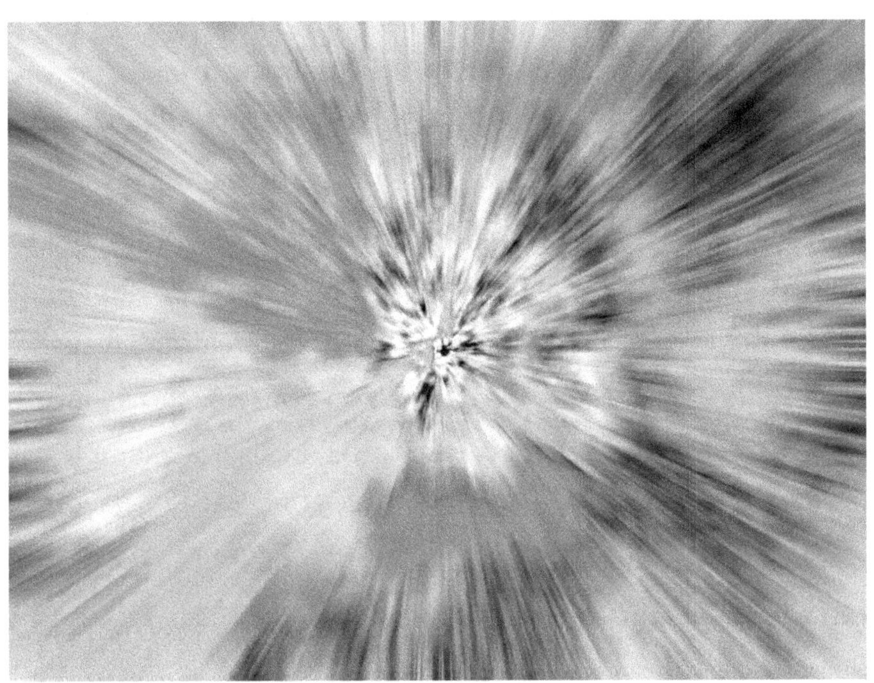

Hypnosis is a state of understanding of focus and concentration. There are two theories about how hypnosis works. The "country" theory implies that subjects enter a different condition of consciousness. The "on-state" concept says that hypnosis isn't an altered state of consciousness. Instead, the topic is responding to a proposal and actively engaging in the semester; instead of under the control of the hypnotist there are hypnosis methods. Among the very common is that the procedure, which entails keeping a constant stare until the eyes shut at a bright object. You're more when you've entered the state of hypnosis suggestible and more inclined to be more amenable to creating changes. Entering into a trance, relaxed state of consciousness Once a trance, the hypnotist will provide verbal ideas, for example, "if you awaken, you will feel more inspired" or even "you won't drink alcohol." Some argue that hypnosis might help recover repressed memories, treat dependence, cure allergies, and decrease depression and anxiety. Hypnosis is focus and responsiveness to tips. You are inclined to be amenable to creating positive behavioral changes.

We actually enter hypnosis each day without even thinking about it. Hypnosis is not like the things we see in Hollywood. You will not be a mindless drone. Nor will you mindlessly follow absurd commands. Instead, you will be able to use hypnosis to improve learning and to embed new lessons into your subconscious mind. Have you ever said to yourself, "I am going to lose weight"? Yet, a few weeks later you realized that you made that decision but still weighed the same, or even more? This is because you made a decision with the conscious mind, the part that is temporal and acts in the moment, rather than the subconscious mind.

In hypnosis, we are precisely the opposite of what Hollywood portrays. Like in meditation, we are more focused, goal-directed, and intuitively aware. Like an old-time cassette tape, you can record over the messages and the negative behavioral patterns of the past. This is why we will not be giving up anything in this first session. As you add new designs and new lessons to your life, you will naturally and intuitively replace old patterns.

There are several new habits that you will add to your life in this first session. First, you will add food to your diet. You will add nutrient-rich foods that are the source of natural energy and health. If you do this each day for a week, you will find that you will effortlessly eat less of the unhealthy things that may have been a part of your life. You will also add a new method of eating. The result will be recording over old patterns that, in the past, have been destructive. You will also add new activities to life and increase your daily physical activity.

The first step is to learn how to enter a state of hypnosis. For beginners, the easiest way to do this is to use guided relaxation.

In fact, because guided relaxation is a great way to manage stress, it will be your first new skill for managing weight. Many of our unhealthy patterns come from emotional reactions to stress. Most people never take the time, like you are doing today, to learn how to practice this skill.

So, by going through this necessary process you will have already added a tool that can be useful to you. Relaxation is a way of entering hypnosis because in a relaxed state we are open to new lessons and are comfortable considering new options. There is no right or wrong way to experience this. Begin by getting comfortable in your chair. In a few minutes, you will be very relaxed. However, you will always be attentive, able to hear my voice, and aware of your surroundings. You might listen to outside noises, but these will not distress you. In fact, they will reassure you that you are exactly where you need to be, doing exactly what you need to be doing.

Now that you have found a comfortable place to still the body and the mind, begin by scanning your body. Anywhere you are carrying the tension of the day in your muscles, simply let those muscles relax. Pay attention to the small muscles of the brow and around the eyes. Let them relax as well. Often, tension is held in tissues of the jaw. You can even allow these muscles to relax. As you relax, notice that you're breathing becomes slower and more natural. As you listen to the quiet in the room or hear the distant sounds of others outside of the room, give yourself permission to enjoy this time of developing a sense of deep relaxation.

As your hands rest on your lap, let them feel very relaxed, very heavy, and very calm. Again, scan your body and relinquish any remaining tension. Relax any residual tension held in the shoulders, back, or legs. Now, notice that your breathing is slower and calm. In just a few moments, your heart rate has even slowed. This necessary process of physical relaxation can also be used to still the mind. Do not worry if your account has been wandering or thinking. After all, this is what brains do. Imagine yourself under a clear blue sky. You can imagine that you are in a place you have been to before, would like to go, or a situation entirely of your own creation. In the sky, there is a single white puffy cloud, gently drifting towards the horizon. As it floats, send all of your thoughts, cares, and concerns into that cloud. Watch the cloud move farther and farther towards the horizon, until it disappears altogether. Now, both your body and mind are completely relaxed. If any other thoughts surface, just allow them to drift towards the horizon after that puffy cloud.

What is Self-Hypnosis?

The only significant difference between hypnosis and self-hypnosis is that in the first one, the operator and the subject are two different people, while in self-hypnosis the operator and the subject coincide in the same person.

This shared experience can be of great value to both, as it will unite them mentally and emotionally and promote love and mutual respect.

It is also a fact that learning is more comfortable and faster when done with another person.

Ask your partner to hypnotize you using a procedure similar to the one we used in the second session. Then practice the self-hypnosis exercise for a few days. Ask your partner once again to hypnotize you and reinforce hypnotic suggestion. Practice it again.

The number of times it is necessary to reinforce the procedure depends entirely on you. If you practice the daily self-hypnosis exercise, one or two reinforcement sessions will be sufficient.

But what about those who have no one with whom to share the learning experience of self-hypnosis? What can they do? How can they learn?

The Sense Spiral

This technique was developed by Betty Erickson, the wife of the famous psychiatrist and hypnotherapist Milton Erickson. It consists of stimulating all sensory perceptions to provoke a saturation (and therefore a relaxation) of the conscious.

First, focus your attention on a specific point at eye level or slightly above it. With your eyes open or closed, start by stating (aloud or in thought) 5 sentences that describe your visual experience ("I see); then five sentences describing your hearing experience ("I hear), then five sentences describing your kinesthetic experience ("I feel...").

Then repeat the same sequence, but with 4 sentences, then 3, then 2, then only one per direction.

Steps to Enable Self-Hypnosis

You would need to feel physically confident and secure to start the cycle. Seek to use a quick calming method.

Choose an item on which you can concentrate your eyes and mind – hopefully, this item would include you gazing upward directly on the wall or ceiling in front of you.

Free your mind of all thoughts and only concentrate on your goal. Obviously, this is hard to do, so take your time and let your emotions leave you.

Become mindful of your pupils, talk of making your eyelids heavy, and shutting gradually. Concentrate on breathing while your eyes shut, breathe in a deep and even manner.

Tell yourself every time you breathe out, you'll relax more. Slow your breathing, and let each breath relax deeper and deeper.

Use your mind's eye to visualize a gentle movement of an object up and down or sideways. Maybe a metronome's hand or a pendulum-something that has a normal, long, yet steady movement. See the object sway back and forth in your mind's eye or up and down.

Softly, gradually and monotonously start the countdown from ten in your mind, saying after each count, 10 I'm relaxing. '9 I'm calming etc.

Believe, and remember that you will have reached your hypnotic state when you finish counting down.

It is the time when you enter the hypnotic condition to reflect on the specific messages you've written. Focus on each statement-see it in the eye of your mind, repeat it in your thoughts. Relax and keep focused.

Relax and clear your mind before getting out of your hypnotic state once again.

Count steadily but energetically to 10. Reverse the process you used when you were counting down to your hypnotic state before. Use some positive messages, as you count, between every number. '1, I'll feel like I've had a full night' sleep when I wake up'... etc.

When you hit 10 you feel fully awakened and reborn! Let your conscious mind slowly catch up with the day's events and continue to feel refreshed.

Leave your worries aside.

It is possible to use self-hypnosis to solve virtually any type of problem and also to broaden your consciousness and connect with your innate superior intelligence and creative ability. By using self-hypnosis for the latter purpose, hypnosis can be transformed into meditation.

Self-hypnosis can also be used in those moments when you feel the need for a higher power to intervene in some situations; then, it becomes a prayer. The subtle differences between these forms of self-hypnosis lie in the way thoughts are guided once the state of consciousness itself has been altered, that is when the alpha state has been reached.

What a fantastic tool is self-hypnosis! It transports us to another state while we are comfortably and quietly sitting with our eyes closed, thinking about a specific objective. But using self-hypnosis in this sense is not easy to achieve since it requires a prolonged period of preconditioning in a hypnotic or auto hypnotic state. Such preconditioning is similar to that used for diet control, but the indications are different; it will be necessary to devise the techniques and suggestions for this case.

And it also requires practice, a lot of practice. Do not forget my words, time and effort will be rewarded with the results. Develop your discipline and stick to it; the results will be a real success.

Hypnosis for Weight Loss

In terms of weight loss, you already know the standard professionals: doctors, dietitians, personal trainers, and even psychological state coaches. But maybe you haven't thought of a hypnotist yet. Facts have proven that the utilization of hypnosis is different, and people take risks in weight loss. Greg Gorniak, a clinical and medical hypnotist, practicing in Ontario, said that sometimes, all other final efforts are tried and failed before it can pass.

But it's not that others control their thinking and let themselves do some exciting things in a comatose state. Kimberly Friedmutter, a hypnotherapist and author of Subscious Power, said: "Mind control, which is against your will, is the biggest misunderstanding of hypnosis." Due to how the show business portrays hypnotists, people are pleased to ascertain that I'm not wearing a black robe or swinging my watch from a sequence."

Can Hypnosis Help Lose Weight?

According to Malian Colman, the chairman of the Australian Association of Hypnotherapists (AHA), hypnosis can bring good results to customers trying to find weight loss assistance. However, she acknowledged that the virtual circle belt isn't for everybody. "(Virtual circle belt) works well in some people, but weight loss is complicated, and people's motivations for eating or overeating could also be very different. The therapist will work with the client to spot the matter for excellent hypnosis."

Lyndall Briggs, president of the Australian Association of Clinical Hypnotherapists (ASCH), said that she has been using hypnosis to scale back her clients' load over the years and has succeeded in hypnosis treatment. Still, she believes that a size suitable for all treatments isn't a fair idea. She said: "Different methods serve different customers."

Professor Clare Collins, a spokesperson for the Australian Association of Nutritionists (DAA), said that surprisingly. There are few studies on hypnosis and weight loss, which she attributed to "the disconnect between science and practice." She noted that past research results are mixed and difficult to realize because you can't blindly test subjects.

She added that a comprehensive review published in 2014 by Liverpool John Moores University reviewed previous research and results. The study's entire finding is by combining hypnotic drugs with traditional weight management strategies and using them continuously (rather than one time), some people enjoy hypnosis. However, the review found that anesthesia isn't valid for everybody, and hypnosis is considered to favor only those who are willing to accept advice.

Collins said that hypnosis could affect negative self-talk and shortcut self-destruction in the diet for those that respond well;

it can help overweight people become symptoms of past trauma. Collins emphasized that before all folks rushed so far, hypnosis alone was never enough. "There could also be other cognitive-behavioral therapies that are more suitable for a few individuals than other individuals (hypnosis), know what a healthy diet is, change eating habits, and exercise. You cannot just place your hopes on hypnosis."

Surprisingly, many scientific studies specialize in the effect of hypnosis on weight loss, many of which are positive. Original research completed in 1986 found that overweight women using hypnosis procedures lost 17 pounds, while women who had to concentrate on the diet lost 0.5 pounds. In the 1990s, a meta-analysis of hypnotic weight loss found that subjects who used hypnosis lost twice the maximum amount of weight as those that didn't. A 2014 study found that ladies using hypnotic drugs can improve body weight, BMI, eating behavior, and even improve body image.

But this is often not good news: A 2012 Stanford University study found that a few quarters of individuals couldn't hypnotize in the least. Contrary to popular belief, it had nothing to do with their personality. On the contrary, some people's brains don't seem to figure that way. "If you're tough to daydream, often hooked into books or watching movies, and do not think you're creative, then you'll be one among the people with poor hypnosis," Dr. Stan said. Georgia said that this not only helped her lose excess weight but also helped her maintain her weight. Six years later, she was happily maintaining weight loss, and infrequently checked again with a hypnotist therapist.

Who Should Try Hypnosis to Lose Weight?

The perfect candidates are those that enforce a healthy diet and exercise plan because they can't obviate bad habits. He said that stepping into bad habits (such as eating an entire bag of potato chips rather than stopping once you are full) may be a sign of a mental problem.

Friedman says that your subconscious mind is where your emotions, habits, and addiction are. Moreover, since hypnosis is aimed toward conscious people and unconscious people, it's going to be simpler.

Research analysis from 1970 found that hypnosis's success rate reached 93%, requiring less treatment than psychological and behavioral therapy. "This leads researchers to believe that hypnosis is the best method for changing habits, ways of thinking, and behavior," Friedmutter said. Hypnosis therapy doesn't need to be used alone.

What Do I Expect In Treatment?

The meeting time and method may vary, counting on the doctor. For instance, Dr. Cruz said that her treatment usually lasts 45 to 60 minutes, while Friedman believes that weight loss patients need 3 to 4 hours. But generally, you'll lie down, close your eyes and relax, and let the hypnotherapist guide you through specific skills and suggestions which will assist you in achieving your goals.

Friedman said: "The idea is to coach people to maneuver in a healthy direction but from an unhealthy direction." I used to be ready to identify mental obstacles that caused the customer to interrupt faraway from their [health] original blueprint through the customer's history. Even as we learn to abuse our bodies with food, we will learn to respect them. "No, you'll not giggle sort of a chicken, nor will you confess any profound secrets." Gorniak said: "You can't fall under a hypnotic state or be told or do something against your will." "If it violates your values or beliefs, you'll not take actions that supported the knowledge provided during the trance."

Gorniak added that, on the contrary, you'll feel deeply relaxed while still knowing what you're talking about. He said: "People in a hypnotic state will describe it as between awake and deeply asleep." "They are fully controlled and may stop the method at any time because you'll hypnotize once you prefer to do so. Teamwork to realize personal goals." In fact, the number of coaching sessions required depends entirely on your response to hypnosis. Dr. Cruz said that some people might only see one to three results, while others may have eight to fifteen meetings. Again, it's not going to work for everybody.

How Does Hypnosis Feel?

Forget everything you see in movies and on stage; therapeutic hypnosis is closer to healing than circus tricks. Dr. Stan said: "Hypnotherapy is a collaborative experience, and patients should understand things and feel comfortable at every step." For those that are worried about being deceived into doing strange or harmful things, she added, even under hypnosis, if you do not want to do something, you will not roll in the hay either. She explained: "It's just concentration." "Everyone will naturally enter a light state several times a day—think about it once you are planning the world when your friends share every detail of the vacation. Hypnosis is simply learning to require a useful way to focus your attention." Georgia has eliminated hypnosis's parable that makes people feel weird or scared from their patients' perspectives. She says she is usually sober and controlled. There are some exciting moments when to be told to tread on the size and see her target weight visually. "My creative mind must first imagine all clothes, jewelry, watches, and hairpins before beginning. Is anyone else doing this, or is it just me?" (No, not just you, Georgia!)

Ways to Lose Weight

Close your eyes. Imagine your food cravings. Imagine eating what good for you each day is. Imagine that hypnosis can assist you to reduce because the news is: indeed. Jean Fain, a psychotherapist at Harvard school of medicine, has provided you with ten sorts of hypnosis suggestions; please try it now. Once I tell people how I make a living by making a living (as a hypnotist and as a psychotherapist), they're going to ask: Does this work inevitably? My answer usually brightens their eyes between excitement and doubt.

Hypnosis is already available centuries before carbohydrate and calorie counting, but this ancient concentration technique has not been accepted wholeheartedly as an efficient weight-loss strategy. Until recently, there was little scientific evidence to support the legitimate claims of respected hypnosis therapists. Therefore, the massive commitment of their problem (stage hypnotists) didn't play any role.

Unless hypnosis causes you to or someone you recognize happy to shop for a replacement or smaller wardrobe, it's going to be hard to trust that this body-centric approach can help you control your diet.

So, take a glance at yourself. You do not need to bother finding some valuable lessons that hypnosis must teach you to reduce. Subsequent ten mini concepts include some weight loss methods that my weight management clients received during collective and individual hypnosis treatments.

The solution is inside. The hypnotherapist believes you've got everything you would need to succeed. You do not need other nutriment or the newest appetite suppressants. To reduce in weight is to believe your aptitude, just like riding a bicycle; at first, you will have a horrible experience as a first-timer, but you've got to keep practicing until you can automatically ride diligently. Losing weight seems to be beyond your scope, but it's just a matter of finding balance.

Believe it's to ascertain. People tend to realize what they think are often made; it even applies to hypnosis. The themes tricked them into thinking that they might hypnotize (for example, when the hypnotist suggested that they are angered, he turns on the hidden red bulb off) to prove the improved hypnotic response. The expectation of getting assistance is crucial.

If you imagine it, it'll come. Even as athletes steel themselves against the sport, visualizing victory can prepare you for the truth of success. Imagine a healthy diet each day, which will help you imagine the required steps to become a healthy dieter. Is it challenging to portray? Find an old photo of yourself, of moderate weight, and remember what you probably did differently at that time; imagine reviving those routines, or get advice visually from an older, smarter self which reaches the specified weight in the future.

Two strategies are better than one. In terms of weight loss and maintaining weight loss, the successful combination is hypnosis and cognitive-behavioral therapy (CBT), enhancing counterproductive thoughts and behaviors. Customers who have learned these two methods have lost twice their weight without falling into a dieter's disorder and regaining the trap. If you've ever written a food diary, you've already tried CBT. Before my clients learn hypnosis, they're going to track everything after every week or two. Every ethical hypnotherapist knows that raising awareness may be a crucial step towards lasting change.

Whether you wish or not, it's the way of life for the fattest person. There's no suggestion that there's enough power to exceed the survival instinct. It's the survival method; in the case of famine, we still program to survive the fittest. An honest example: a starving diet personal trainer who asked me to advise her to stop the jelly bear addiction. I attempted to elucidate that her body only believes that her life depends on chewy candies. She is not going to hand over the sweets until she has enough calories from more nutritious food. No, she insisted that she only needed one suggestion. I used to be unsurprised when she dropped out of the faculty.

Practice makes perfect. A Pilates session doesn't produce rubbing abs, and a hypnotic exercise doesn't improve diet. However, repeating 15 to twenty minutes of positive advice silently a day can change your eating habits, especially when combined with slow and natural breathing. It's the idea of any behavioral change plan.

Control craving. What if you'll get obviate cravings? Isolate them and send them out? Some weight loss hypnosis techniques can assist you to do that. For instance, you'll be asked to visually send your desires—like the case of a ship going on a bent sea. Recommendations also can assist you in reconstructing your desires and finding out how to manage them more effectively.

Looking forward to success. Expectations determine reality. Once we expect success, we naturally tend to require the required steps to realize success. Weight loss hypnosis can implant fruitful seeds in your brain, becoming a mighty unconscious power to help you stay in a healthy state.

Enthusiasm for practice. Negative factors often destroy weight loss. There are some foods that you "cannot" eat. Unhealthy food is "killing" you. Hypnosis therapy allows us to reimagine these suggestions with a more positive attitude—you won't lose yourself due to this; you're discarding what you do not need.

Able to relapse. We train to think that relapse is that shameful—the reason for abandoning. But hypnosis requires us to believe declines in several ways. Recurrence becomes a chance to see errors, learn from them, and steel oneself against temptation. Modify your behavior. A little step at a time can make big goals. Hypnosis therapy allows us to make small changes to realize larger goals. Suppose you reward yourself with sugary, high-calorie foods; through hypnosis, you'll choose healthier rewards.

Visualization success. Finally, hypnosis visualization may be a powerful motivation. The display allows you to "view" the results and explore how to cause you to feel. You'll also visualize your future self and tell yourself that you simply have everything you would need to succeed.

Congratulations, this is often a relapse. When customers find themselves over-indulging against their healthiest intentions, I congratulate them. Hypnosis treats regression as a chance, not a trivial matter. You'll be better prepared for the inevitable temptations in life if you'll learn from real or imagined relapses

Learn Self-hypnosis to Lead a Better Life

Wonder if you should practice hypnosis of yourself, or is it possible at all? Many people freak out when I mention they are supposed to learn the techniques of hypnosis, not even knowing what self-hypnosis is and how it can benefit their lives in several ways.

We are often witnesses to many serious problems in today 's fast lives, such as stress, time management and all kinds of mental disorders that people experience. We don't even know in most situations that we have some sort of problem in our mind, we just believe it's a temporary state of discomfort or nervousness that will pass by itself. Okay, they won't.

What about all the bad habits and personality traits we have developed over time? Smoking, over-eating, nail-biting, drinking, drug abuse, panic attacks, anxiety, social phobias, shyness, social life withdrawal, insomnia, lack of self-confidence, blushing, stuttering, binge eating, depression, anger, powerlessness ... And the list just keeps going on. The majority of people at any point in their lives will experience at least some of the above conditions.

That's why learning some techniques to clear up all the mess in your mind is essential to your overall well-being, and yesterday you should have started!

Your hands and teeth are typically washed many times a day, but how often do you clean your mind and soul? Have you already learned a method for doing it effectively?

There are many ways to relax and touch the subconscious mind to reprogram and alter it positively, and my personal opinion that one of the best ways to do this is to practice self-hypnosis. Once you master the technique, it won't take you more than 10-15 minutes a day to work on yourself to reach the ultimate goal, regardless of whether it's just to quit smoking or solve a lot of other issues.

It is not difficult to learn the essentials of self-hypnosis, and there is really no need to fear it.

The evidence for this is that over 500 million people are doing it every day around the world to get a better, healthier life.

Self-hypnosis is a state of mind, in which:

Extreme relaxation can happen

You pay special attention to the recommendations you want to bring into action

And helps you to acknowledge and not condemn the suggestions made.

Self-hypnosis helps you to program your subconscious directly with optimistic affirmations and helpful feedback and is a very successful way to alleviate and control stress and promotes deep relaxation in recovery.

Here we shall look at questions such as:

- When can I hypnosis myself practice?

- Where is self-hypnosis best practiced?

- How long am I supposed to practice self-hypnosis?

- Am I in a safe place to lay down or sit down?

- Will I need to close my eyes?

- Personal transition, what could I have expected?

- Is it possible to make the process some time easier?

When can I hypnosis myself practice?

Whenever you have a few minutes free from interruption, disruption or distraction, you can quite easily practice self-hypnosis. Nevertheless, you should never practice while driving, operating or working with any sort of machinery under any conditions whatsoever or while performing any other operation, task or process requiring your full and undivided attention.

Where is self-hypnosis best practiced?

Somewhere secure, clean, relaxed and quiet anywhere would be an ideal place for self-hypnosis practice. Usually indoors, though practicing self-hypnosis nearly anywhere is just as feasible.

If you ensure you can relax, feel relaxed and safe from as much external noise, discomfort or interference as possible, you can achieve more.

How long am I supposed to practice self-hypnosis?

Quality over quantity-as a guide 15 to 20 uninterrupted minutes of quality a day is more significant than 30 to 60 minutes of disturbance and disruption. Set aside a designated time when you are not going to be disturbed.

Keep in mind that all the time you invest in self-hypnosis will be reimbursed as you make a positive, life-affirming change about yourself. Train often as you become more professional you will definitely find that the time you need to train is will.

Am I in a safe place to lay down or sit down?

I achieve your self-hypnotic goal(s) by far more importantly being comfortable. Doing what you feel is most natural will work best and yield better results. Lying down to practice self-hypnosis might make drifting off to sleep too easy for you but if your ultimate goal is to fall to sleep then lying down would be fine.

Once again, many people find that sitting in a calm, supportive position with the assisted head provides the results they need.

Will I need to close my eyes?

Most people skilled in self-hypnosis can quickly and easily go into a trance with their eyes open, but most people feel more comfortable and would find it easier to start with eyes closed.

Personal transition, what could I have expected?

The outcomes you receive will be based solely on the suggestions you make during your self-hypnosis session. You can expect to make meaningful improvements to life, it's perfectly normal to expect the change that will improve your life. Transition is a normal part of our life; it happens to us and all those around us each and every day.

Is it possible to make the process some time easier?

Give yourself a suggestion that you will enter trance faster and easier next time during your self-hypnosis session. In a trance, an example may be: "I can easily return to this profoundly relaxed and concentrated state of consciousness whenever I want, simply by taking a few deep and calming breaths."

Self-Hypnosis - Practical Applications

How can you develop a self-disciplined cast iron and a strong will to succeed? With Self-hypnosis-

Convenient use

If for whatever reason, you do not already have good discipline, what could be the best way to acquire it quickly and effectively?

Every time you practice self-hypnosis, you'll experience a new burst of directional energy and commitment. When you observe what is happening every day in your life, you will constantly find that you are:

- Focus more on the personal and professional objectives

- Learn not to heed those times of self-doubt

- Break down procrastination, become a 'go-getter'

- Creating and sustaining a 'can do' mentality

- Achieve a greater sense of contentment and self-worth

How to practice Hypnosis of yourself

Find a place that is relaxed and quiet and sit down somewhere.

Relax your body by closing your eyes, and imagine relaxing waves running from your scalp down to your toes.

Feel the muscles relaxing in your body as relaxation waves wash them over.

Use suggestions to deepen a relaxing state. This can be as easy as saying: "I feel confident and comfortable with myself. I get more relaxed and comfortable with every step ..."

Use the affirmation(s) you want to install after you feel completely relaxed, you can mix these in with the suggestions for relaxation.

Self-hypnosis is an effective and practical technique for deep relaxation. It can be used with affirmations or without them, depending on what you want to achieve.

Find a comfortable and quiet place to sit down somewhere to use the technique. Think about it and plan, any comments you might want to make. Start with your eyes closed and your muscles relaxed. Using imagery is one good way to do this. Go ahead and use suggestions to relax even more. Using whatever affirmations, you have prepared when you feel really comfortable. Achieve hypnosis status for as long as you like.

CHAPTER 5:

Habits for Weight Loss

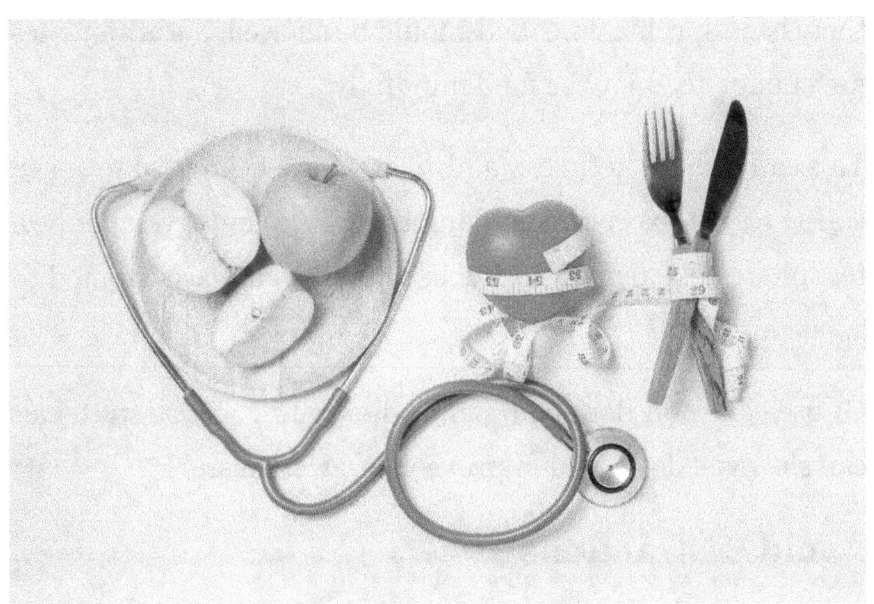

Take Things Slowly

Eating should not be treated as a race. Eat slowly. This just means that you should take your time in relishing and enjoying your food – it is a healthy thing! So, how long do you have to grind up the food in your mouth? Well, there is no specific time food should be chewed, but 18-25 bites are enough to enjoy the food mindfully.

This can be hard at first, mainly if you have been used to speed eating for an exceptionally long time. Why not try some new techniques like using chopsticks when you are accustomed to spoon and fork?

Or use your non-dominant hand when eating. These strategies can slow you down and improve your awareness.

Avoid Distractions

To make things simpler for you, just make it a habit of sitting down and staying away from distractions. The handful of nuts that you eat as you walk through the kitchen and the bunch of morning snacks you nibbled while standing in front of your fridge can be hard to recall.

According to researchers, people tend to eat more when they are doing other things too. You should, therefore, sit down and focus on your food to prevent mindless eating behaviors.

Savor Every Bite

Do not forget that eating mindfully is not only about enjoying the food you eat, but your health too, and without feeling guilty and uncomfortable. Relishing the sight, taste, and smell of your diet is utterly worth it. This can be so easy if you take things gradually and do not rush to perfection. Make small changes towards awareness until you are a fully mindful eater. So, eat slowly and savor the good food you are eating and the proper nutrition you are giving to your body.

Mind the Presentation

Regardless of how busy you are; it is a good idea to set the table – making sure it looks divine. A lovely set of utensils, placement, and napkin made of eco-friendly cloth material is a perfect reminder that you need to sit down and pay attention when you have your meals.

Plate Your Food

Serving yourself and portioning your food before you bring the plate to the table can help you to consume a modest amount, rather than putting a platter on the table from which to replenish continually. You can do this even with crackers, chips, nuts, and other snack foods. Keep yourself away from the temptation of eating straight from a bag of chips and different types of food. It is also helpful if you resize the bag or place the food in smaller containers so that you can stay aware of the amount of food you are eating. Having a bright idea of how much you have eaten will make you stop eating when you are full, or even sooner.

Always Choose Quality over Quantity

By trying to select smaller amounts of the most beautiful food within your means, you will end up enjoying and feeling satisfied without the chance of overeating. With this, it will be helpful if you spend time preparing your meals using quality and fresh ingredients. Cooking can be a pleasurable and relaxing experience if you only let yourself into it. On top of this, you can achieve the peace of mind that comes from knowing what is in the food you are eating.

Do Not Invite Your Thoughts and Emotions to Dinner

Just as there are many other factors that affect our sense of mindful eating, as well as the digestive system; it would come as no surprise that our thoughts and emotions play just as much of an important role.

It happens on the odd occasion that one comes home after a long and tiresome day and you feel somewhat "worked up," irritated and angry. This is when negative and even destructive thoughts creep in while you are having supper.

The best practice would be to avoid this altogether. Therefore, if you are feeling unhappy or angry in any way, go for a walk before supper, play with your children, or play with your family pet. But, whatever you do, take your mind off your negative emotions, before you attempt to have a meal.

Make a Good Meal Plan for Each Week

When you start the diet, it is advised to stick to the meal plan that comes with the diet. There should be a meal plan of 2 weeks or 4 weeks attached to the diet's guideline. Once you are familiar with the food list, prohibited ingredients, cooking techniques and how to go grocery shopping for your diet, it will be easier for you to twist and change things in the meal plan. Do not try to change the meal plan for the first 2 weeks. Stick to the meal plan they give you. If you try to change it right at the beginning, you may feel lost or feel terrified in the beginning. So, it is advised to try and introduce new recipes and ideas after you are 2 weeks into the diet.

Drink Lots of Water

Staying hydrated is the key to living a healthy life in general. It is not relevant for only diets, but in general we should always be drinking enough water to keep ourselves hydrated. Dehydration can bring forth many unwanted diseases. When you are dehydrated, you feel very dizzy, lightheaded, nauseous, and lethargic. You cannot focus on anything well. Urinary infection occurs, which triggers other health issues.

Being on a diet, the purpose of drinking water is to help you process the different food you are eating and to help digest it well. Water helps in proper digestion; it helps in extracting bad minerals from our body. Water also gives us a glow on the skin.

Never Skip Breakfast

It is essential to eat a full breakfast to keep yourself moving actively throughout the day. It gives you a great boost, good metabolism and your digestion starts properly functioning during the day. When you skip breakfast, everything sort of disrupts. Your day starts slow and soon you would feel restless. It is especially important to have a good meal at the beginning of your day in order to be productive for the rest of the day.

If you are terribly busy, try to have your breakfast on the go. Grab breakfast in a box or a mason jar and have it in the car or on the bus or whatever transport you are using to get to your work. You can also have your breakfast at a healthy restaurant where they serve food that is in sync with your diet.

Eat Protein

Protein is particularly good for the body. It helps your brain function better. Protein can come from both animal and non-animal products. So even if you are a vegetable or vegan, you can still enjoy your protein from plants. Soy, mushroom, legumes, and nuts are a few examples. Eating protein keeps you strong and healthy. Eating protein increases your brain function. On the other hand, if you do not eat enough protein for the day, your entire way would be wasted. You will not be able to focus on anything properly. You would feel dizzy and weak all through the day. If you are a vegetarian, or vegan you can enjoy avocado, coconut, almond, cashew, soy, and mushroom to get protein.

Eat Super Foods

Most people eat foods that do not necessarily affect them in the best way. Where some foods may enhance some people's energy levels, it may impact others more negatively. The important thing is to know your food. It may be a good idea to keep a food journal, and if you know that certain foods affect you negatively, one should try to avoid those foods and stick to healthier options. It is a fact that most people enjoy foods which they should probably not be eating. However, if you wish to eat mindfully and enhance your health and a general sense of wellbeing, then it would be best to eat foods that will precisely do that.

There are also various foods that are classified as superfoods. These would include your lean and purest sources of protein, such as free-range chicken, as well as a variety of fresh fruit, vegetable, and herbs.

Stop Multitasking While You Eat

Multitasking is defined as the simultaneous execution of more than one activity at one time. Though it is a skill that we should master, often it leads to unproductive activity. The development of our economy leads to a more hectic way of living. Most of us develop the habit of doing one thing while doing another. This is true even when it comes to eating.

Smaller Plates, Taller Glasses

This habit changer ties in a little bit with drinking more water; however, it is a bit different. People tend to fill up their plates with food, so the size of the plate matters. If you have a large plate, you are going to put more food on your plate but, if you have a smaller plate, you will have less food on your plate.

Stay Positive

The secret to succeeding in anything is being positive. When you start something new, always stay positive regarding it. You need to keep a positive mind, an open mind rather. You cannot be anxious, hasty, and restless in a diet. You need to keep calm and do everything that calms you down. Overthinking can lead to being bored and not interested in the diet very soon. The power of positivity is immense. It cannot be compared with anything else.

On the other hand, when you start something with a negative mindset, it eventually does not work out. You end up leaving it behind or failing at it because you had doubts right at the beginning. A doubtful mind cannot focus properly, and the best never comes out from a doubtful mind.

Eating mindlessly can cause anyone to eat way too much and this is what happens to most of us. The problem is that when people are eating, they are hardly thinking about what they are doing. Instead, their minds are on other things and this leads them not to be aware of how much they are eating.

Beware of the portions.

Many individuals eat approximately twice the average amount of meals consumed. Restaurants also deliver large servings, which will teach your mind to believe that the quantity of food the body requires is not beneficial to have hands-on the right serving proportions

Put the spoon down in between the bites.

It forces you to eat more gradually, which would be an easy calorie-cutting strategy. Whenever you take your time rather than snorting your meals, your body will naturally enroll the feeling of satiety that can take approximately 20 minutes to signal your brain. Plus, gradually eating will help the food to taste even better.

Gulp down water 24/7.

Although the body is basically a fairly smart tool, it can be vulnerable to slip-ups. "Sometimes, it is dehydration that triggers what you believe is a hunger pang. The" hunger "will lead you to snack because all your body requires would be some water.

Taking some time out to make lunch.

Not only can you save time by cooking your own lunch, but it can also make sure you exactly realize what you're putting in your body, so you get the correct foods. You're still less prone to miss lunch on busy days because you can only walk to the supermarket instead of trying to run out to purchase food. While missing those meals could help improve weight reduction, trying to deprive your body of regular meals will make you more likely to overeat it later.

Do not do anything else whilst you eat.

Focusing on food while there's stuff to do and viewing Instagram may be difficult, but munching away while you're disturbed will lead you to unintentionally indulge with more than you should. Disturbed food doesn't only create further intake at the time; it can also force you to consume further later in the day than is required.

Emphasize breakfasts.

"Eating a meal packed with healthy fiber and protein should keep you satiated, and will help you make healthier food decisions every day. Choose meals that are not carbohydrate explosions without something significant to hold you full, such as hash browns, warm cereal, and croissants, to maximize breakfast power. "Try poached eggs on the whole grain toast, simple Greek yogurt with a bowl of your preferred fruit, or a veggie-laden omelet.

Be clever when snacking.

If you're attempting to lose weight, snacking may be either your best friend or a potentially supportive, but undoubtedly manipulative saboteur. There's the problem of unknowingly getting in more than you thought, which you can remedy in a snap by pre-portioning the treats as per their portion sizes instead of only gnawing away at them willy-nilly. Another issue with snacking can arise if you eat without check throughout the day, rather than snacking mindfully. Check out the snacking habits for weight loss tips to make sure you are on the right path.

Sleep through adequate hours each night.

It may be tough to adhere to a healthy sleep schedule — especially while there are episodes of serial to catch up on — but having adequate rest is an effective way to promote weight loss. Sleeping helps maintain the hunger hormones leptin and ghrelin in control. Without an appropriate quantity, those hormones get unbalanced and may contribute to increased appetite.

Keep eating healthy as well on Sundays.

If you're infatuated with having eaten possibly the best Monday through Friday but consider weekends an unrestricted-for-all food, you might not see the weight loss you're hoping for.

If you add it all up, trying to eat poorly and not exercising Friday through Sunday tends to come out to 12 days off a month.

Instead of allowing weekdays to impact your habits, focus on achieving a positive lifestyle — with the occasional treat — that's feasible.

Concentrate upon small plates.

If you look at the same amount of food on a tiny plate vs. a big one, your eyes could tell you there's even more awesomeness on the smaller plate. Even though you don't consume enough, cutting down on the amount of plate area surrounding your food will drip your mind.

However, doing its opposite may trigger your appetite by forcing you to think you only ate a little bit.

Scale back on eating in family style.

When you dine with serving dishes full of extra help right in front of you, you can slip into refilling your plate carelessly even if you're not still hungry. Instead, if feasible, restrict the meal on the table about what you have to eat. This is not to conclude seconds are strictly prohibited — just review in and see if you're still starving prior to actually getting back to reach a little more.

In restaurants, the seat faced away from the buffet table.

Seeing more food in your sightline will drive you into food-coma territory, particularly if you're trying to maximize the benefit of your money. Instead of eating when thinking about what you can reward yourself with next, turn your attention to the other food, and concentrate on just embracing what's on your dish. If you'd like more food once you're finished, the buffet would still be there.

Place vegetables up on the plate.

One of the easiest strategies to fall into a healthier eating routine is by introducing foods to the diet rather than cutting them. Failing to consume all of the beloved snacks will go end up backfiring in a spree, whereas gradually raising your food consumption will only produce positive results. "Not only are veggies packed with essential nutrients to keep the body balanced and energized, but they also provide fiber to makes you lean. Beginning small to prevent vegetable burnout: add a cup of them just to at most one meal per day for a week and continue to integrate them into even more foods once you get accustomed to them.

Keep a diary of food.

If you practice any of these, but you don't see any significant weight reduction, it may seem like a complicated problem you really can't break. Keep a diet diary in any situation, such that you'll have a thorough and overall image of your behaviors. "It will help you identify places that are unique to both you and the habits that might use a little adjustment. Do the utmost and maintain control with the food and drink consumption for a whole week and check out and see whether you are unintentionally getting in a few additional calories that you should leave out and achieve the results you are seeking. Note, above all, that losing the weight always requires certain experimentation — but the idea is this is a long way you're practicing how to be healthy with the fitness, which really counts.

CHAPTER 6:

Benefits of Intuitive Eating

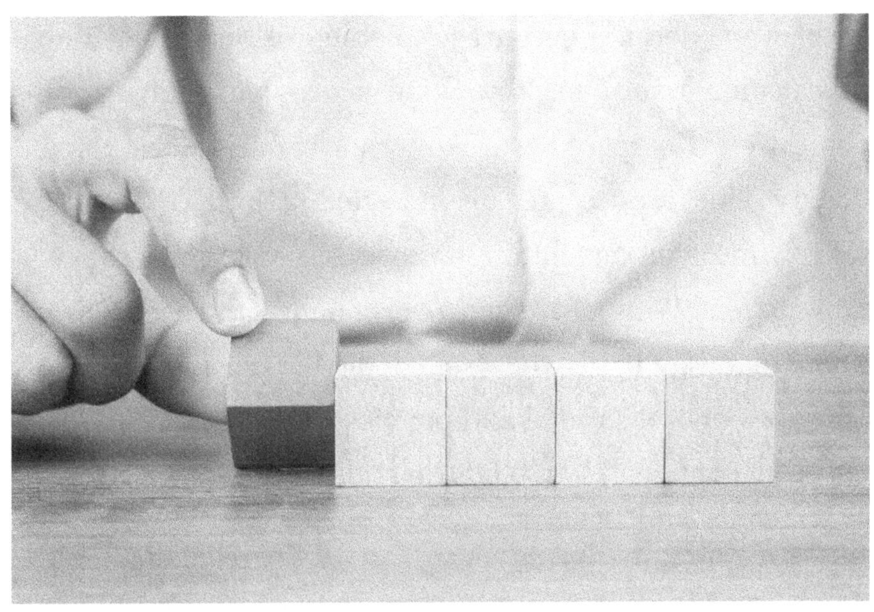

Intuitive eating is a non-diet approach, mind, and body approach to wellness and health. This approach doesn't encourage dieting but emphasizes taking note of the inner body and hunger cues. By trusting our bodies, intuitive healing renews our relationship with food.

Though it doesn't encourage dieting, it uses nutritional information to form healthy eating choices and habits. By this habit, we eat because we'd like to not because we've to, and dietary values are accepted disinterestedly. During this method, we rely more on our intuition. Food is employed to satisfy a requirement. Without the inner cue of hunger, no need for food. Those that want to flee the strain of dieting can appreciate this approach since it's useful and practical. There's no connection between emotions and food during this sort of eating.

Intuitive eating is not intended for weight reduction. Sadly, there might be dietitians, mentors, and different experts that sell intuitive eating as a diet, which runs counter to the thought altogether. The objective of intuitive eating is improving your association with food. This incorporates building more beneficial food practices and trying not to control the scale. That being stated, pretty much everyone experiencing the way toward figuring out how to be an intuitive eater needs to get thinner—else, they would as of now be intuitive eaters!

Intuitive eating enables your body to break the diet cycle and sink into its regular set point weight territory. This might be lower, higher, or a similar weight you are at present.

How Intuitive Eating Plays a Role in Healthy Living and Shopping Lifestyle:

Intuitive eating guides our lives inside and out. It creates such a lot of opportunity and straightforwardness by not stressing over what I will eat or when I will eat it. I stream with what my body guides me to eat, and when it guides me to it eat-and with that, it creates opportunity inside my relationship in my body and how I feel about myself. I am more advantageous and more adjusted than I have ever been in my body and I can say that I love my body and this vessel that I am carrying on with this life in. This move-in my association with my body, food and my general surroundings is an immediate consequence of my otherworldly voyage.

The most significant thing is to not stress over the 'right' or 'wrong' choice, and instead to distinguish how you are feeling and where in your body you think it-with the goal that you aren't eating to keep away from or conceal feelings. That way, your eating decisions are simpler to make since they are not enveloped with your passing feelings.

There is such a lot of opportunity and facilitate that shows up when you interface with and pursue your instinct. Shopping for food turns out to be, to a lesser degree a task or a problem and increasingly an action of happiness and articulation. To have the option to purchase what looks, sounds, and scents great (offers to the faculties) and to believe my instinct as far as what I will cook and create each day/week. It additionally makes the creation procedure progressively fun since you do not feel adhered to pursue a formula or dinner plan. Once more, there is an opportunity. Shopping for food is only an expansion of that and part of the creation procedure (where motivation comes in).

Indeed, there might, in any case, be times when you do not feel like shopping for food or preparing; however, in those minutes, you are not hung up on it. The dread of settling on an inappropriate choice or eating inappropriate food vanishes. Intuitive eating is not about control and dread; it is about the stream and following what feels better (from a space of instinct, not damage or self-hurt).

You are beginning the adventure of understanding what foods reverberate with your body, and what doesn't-interfaces with the act of enthusiastic mindfulness. On the off chance that we shut ourselves off from feeling our feelings, at that point, we are additionally closing our capacity to feel different sensations. Consider it like this-your body is sending you the flag of what feels better and what doesn't; however, you have unplugged the wire association between the inclination, and you are accepting and being informed of the disposition.

Having an essential comprehension of sustenance is a great spot to begin to start to teach oneself and acclimate oneself with specific establishments of pure sciences. From that point, it truly is an act of backing off and carrying your attention to how you feel previously, during and after eating. At whatever point you notice examples of side effects, you should investigate. What musings did you see, how could you feel, what was going on around then? A great deal of our food and eating practices/designs have been adapted and created quite a while prior and requires bringing our cognizance again into that space to develop progressive movements. The most significant piece of this procedure is to curry sympathy with you and practice non-judgment.

The diet culture is a finished square to instinct. It is established in dread and control-and expels the opportunity to interface with how you feel or what your body wants. The diet culture mirrors the longing to change and control the body, instead of helping it and work with it. It is tied in with stifling the body's direction framework (through control), which expels you further away from your instinct and the capacity to interface with your intuition through your body's informing structure. The greatest thing to perceive is that your body is profoundly insightful and realizes what to do-the more that you work with it and backing (and trust it)- the more joyful you will feel.

At whatever point we hop onto a pattern it is imperative to associate with what feels better (and to inquire as to whether this pattern genuinely impacts you or on the off chance that you are merely doing it since others are, and their outcomes entice you). A great spot to ground yourself in what your intuitive direction is, is to ask yourself "What feels useful for your spirit?"

The Health Benefits of Intuitive Eating

<u>There Is No Room for Stress:</u>

Studies have demonstrated that intuitive eaters not just appreciate a more lovely enthusiastic state than dieters, yet additionally experience enhancements in despair, nervousness, negative self-talk, and general mental prosperity when they change to eating intuitively.

The explanation behind this decrease in pressure may originate from the way that when you eat intuitively, you get the chance to concentrate more on making the most of your food as opposed to dissecting it. You additionally remove yourself from the outlook of, "I can't have that since I have to get thinner," or "I can't have carbs because I'm fat."

These sorts of responses to food put a heap of weight at the forefront of your thoughts and body, so it is no big surprise you feel better when you let them go!

Improvement in Digestion:

Two of the fundamental precepts of intuitive eating are to:

- Eat just when you are ravenous,

- Eat until you are fulfilled, not stuffed.

- Rehearsing both propensities can help improve your assimilation in various manners.

For one, eating just when you are genuinely hungry gives your stomach related framework time to discharge your stomach from your last supper. This may appear no major ordeal, and however, when you continue eating each couple of hours and not enabling your food to process, your framework can undoubtedly move toward becoming exhausted. Your stomach needs to consistently siphon out chemicals and acids to help digest your food, while your liver is ceaselessly being attempted to channel poisons and condensation fat.

Additionally, eating until you are full at each feast can shield your assimilation from running comfortably. You are basically "Backing up" your framework by pouring undigested food over half-processed food, which may make you experience acid reflux, stoppage, or any number of stomach related issues.

Rehearsing body mindfulness, eating just until you are fulfilled, and not eating between suppers except if you're eager gives your stomach related framework a rest with the goal that it's completely prepared to deal with your next dinner.

High Self-Esteem:

Notwithstanding improving eating examples and nervousness levels, contemplates have additionally demonstrated that rehearsing intuitive eating develops confidence.

For example, members in a single report experienced more acknowledgment of their bodies and less mental pain concerning their bodies. They were additionally ready to relinquish "Unfortunate weight control practices."

By improving your confidence, it is just typical that different parts of your life will improve too. At the point when you are concentrating less on not being "Sufficient," and more on tolerating yourself, you will generally encounter less nervousness and have an increasingly inspirational point of view. Thus, this can prompt many open doors at work and enhancements in your connections.

A Possibility to Aid Weight Loss:

Studies have likewise indicated that intuitive eaters have lower weight records (BMIs) than dieters. One of the significant purposes behind this could be because of the way that intuitive eating is anything, but difficult to adhere to (not at all like trend diets) which can prompt long haul weight reduction.

At the point when you eat intuitively, you additionally figure out how to regard the satiety flag that discloses to you when you are fulfilled, versus only eating for eating. This outcome is a natural, ideal calorie balance that could prompt weight reduction on the off chance that you have been overeating by disregarding yearning signs.

The way that intuitive eating lessens feelings of anxiety can likewise assume a job since a lot of the pressure hormone cortisol can cause fat addition.

A Decent Improvement In Body Awareness:

Monitoring your body and what it is motioning to you is critical with regards to keeping up your wellbeing. On the off chance that you listen intently, your body will offer you inconspicuous hints that something is not right, enabling you to give it what it needs before it turns into a significant issue.

Take, for instance, indications of supplement inadequacies. Numerous individuals are so separated from their bodies that they do not see unobtrusive signs of a supplement insufficiency, like an absence of vitality or shivering in their grasp and feet. When they do understand, the inadequacy has turned out to be dangerous to such an extent that they need to go to the specialist to get it dealt with.

Intuitive eating is tied in with connecting with your body's sign of craving and satiety. Be that as it may, when you start focusing on these signs, you will begin to be hyper-mindful of different signs your body is emitting. This will enable you to be in line with what you need consistently, so you can deal with it before it turns into an all-out issue.

CHAPTER 7:

Hypnotherapy for weight loss

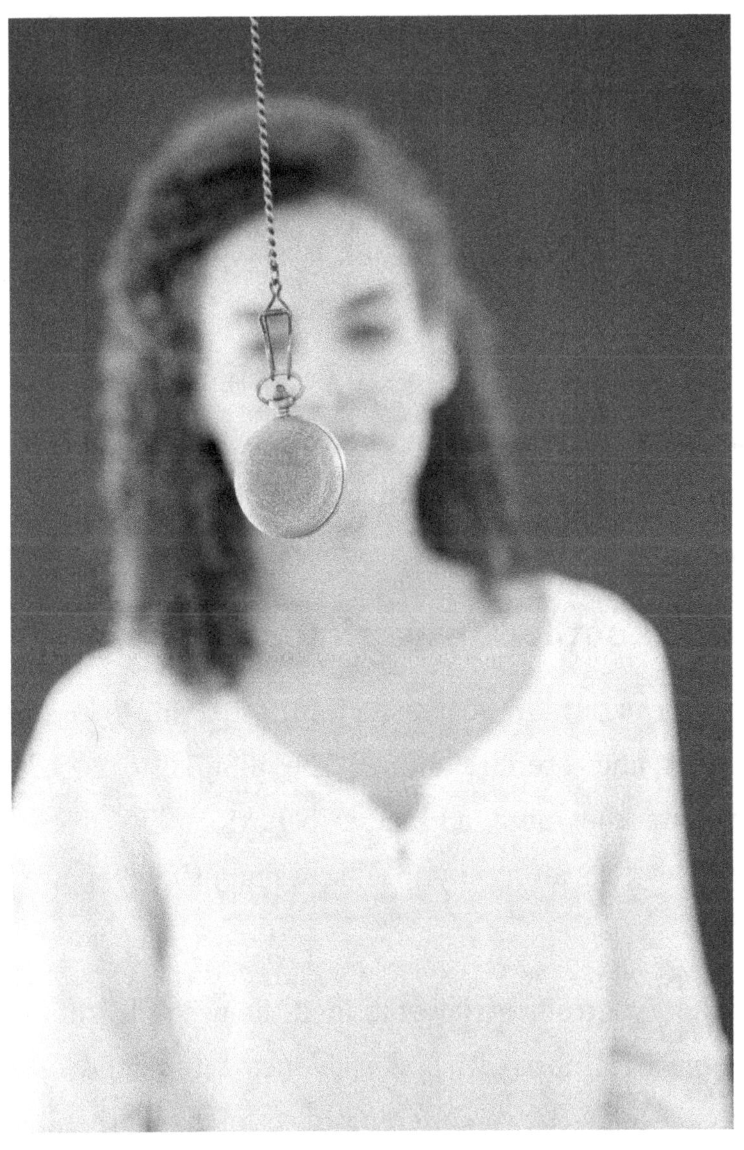

To put oneself in a state of hypnosis, or to make hypnosis with a practitioner, is to intentionally reproduce this state of consciousness with an objective that varies according to the framework in question (relaxation, care, personal development, etc.).

The hypnotic state is the reproduction of a natural and spontaneous state; everyone can have access to it, but not necessarily in the same way. While most individuals respond well to direct verbal suggestions, others will need an indirect approach to bring about the desired altered state of consciousness.

On the other hand, learning the method and its regular repetition allows everyone to be able to enter hypnosis with greater ease and speed: as with a sport, the more you exercise and the more you progress!

Does hypnotherapy work for weight loss?

Hypnosis can be more successful for those trying to lose weight than diet and exercise alone. The aim is to be able to manipulate the mind and alter behaviors like overeating. Nonetheless, it's always up for discussion just how powerful it can be.

An earlier, controlled trial examined the use of hypnotherapy in people with obstructive sleep apnea for weight loss. The research explored two different types of hypnotherapy and basic nutritional recommendations for weight loss and sleep apnea. Within three months, all 60 participants lost 2 to 3 percent of their body weight.

The hypnotherapy participant had shed, on average, an additional 8 pounds at the 18-month follow-up. While this additional loss was not significant, the researchers concluded that hypnotherapy justified more studies as a treatment for obesity. A weight-reduction study that involved hypnotherapy, primarily cognitive-behavioral therapy (CBT), found that this culminated in a slight drop in body weight relative to the placebo community. Researchers have hypothesized that although hypnotherapy can improve weight loss, there is not enough work to persuade them.

It's important to remember that there is not any evidence for weight reduction in favor of hypnosis alone. Most of what you'll learn in conjunction with food and exercise or treatment is in hypnotherapy.

Hypnotherapy Can Aid You to Change Developed Habits through the Power of Hypnosis

Crack the cycle of comfort eating by resolving the issue at the point that it is rooted in the unconscious mind. You can see some important improvements take place over the process of hypnotherapy treatment:

You're becoming more comfortable and your thinking is simpler

Holding the emotional and social needs apart will start to sound normal and therefore inevitably happen

You should search for more innovative ways to channel the thoughts and work with them

The appetite for healthier food will increase and it will significantly boost the diet

You will continue to feel more optimistic, more comfortable, and satisfied with your everyday life without a relentless cross.

Why Hypnotherapy for Losing Weight Can Help You

Have you ever wondered about food as if it were your friend? Have you ever thought that your family and friends are a priority? If you sincerely answer every one of these inquiries, you will come to learn that food is intended to be your companion. You would certainly regard it with greater respect when speaking about it in that manner. Since we just have one body and our health care bill worsens with time, we are most likely expected to take care of ourselves. The same refers to kicking unhealthy habits such as smoking, eating too much alcohol, likely taking mind-altering medications, and also other harmful effects such as sleep deprivation. Hypnosis is all about changing yourself, and you can eventually shift your attitude about diet, exercise, and unhealthy behavior if you will enter a place where you are concentrated on enhancing your health and are able to do so on a regular basis. It would become part of the routine to consume food that is good for your health. Having an ambitious target for yourself, such as completing 21 days of eating healthy, will inevitably lead to all those results if you continue to stick to self-hypnosis. You will build new routines and commonalities for twenty-one days of stability, which will hold you onboard long when you have met your targets for weight loss. Healthy eating after some time will not feel like a penalty, but more like a treat. You'll feel healthier by eating better, but also consuming less If you're like most individuals, you probably enjoy food and eating in general; that doesn't mean that you can't love your meals simply because you practice a diet and exercise schedule. Bearing in mind, though, that you have 3 meals per day, and probably snacks once or twice a day, you should be conscious that not that much food is needed for your body. If the measurement of your both hands clasped together in a fist is the size of your stomach, so where does the majority of the food you eat go? It gets stored as body fat, which is just what you don't like. Concentrate on feeding mindfully and listening to the body. You will also learn that consuming less really leaves you more comfortable. One of the biggest effects of hypnosis promotes your mentality about food and exercise. It changes your mood greatly. While certain individuals who participate in hypnosis use so to monitor their dietary patterns, the sedentary lives of most people are subject to a tone of adjustments. You are a human being, and you are supposed to run, search, and catch. You will rot away and die if you keep sitting all day and don't drive your body out of its comfort bubble.

The work of the hypnotherapist

Generally, the first session begins with an interview with the consultant in order to define his needs, and to determine the approach and methods to be used. This very first session is generally longer than the following and each technique is adapted to the client's needs. A typical session lasts 50 or 60 minutes. Most people start to see results after 4 meetings. Hypnosis is recognized as brief therapy. A dozen meetings are generally sufficient, at least for well-defined problems. In children, usually easier to hypnotize, changes are often seen after only 1 or 2 visits.

How to choose your hypnotherapist?

Don't just rely on word of mouth. It is useful to learn about the internet and to take the time to read the advice and information provided by the practitioner. These are important and allow you to get an idea of his style and approach. You can also call the practitioner to discuss your needs and expectations. It is essential to go to a professional with excellent training in psychotherapy or health, depending on the case to be treated. Ideally, he should know the mechanisms of the problem at hand, whatever it is (physical, psychological, relational, etc.). However, more than the techniques used by a given therapist,

Hypnotherapist, hypnotist, what differences?

The hypnotherapist is a specialist who uses hypnosis in order to treat and support his patient towards well-being, while the hypnotist designates an individual who knows how to bring about the state of hypnosis. While the former must have training and practice in the health sector, the latter is more active in the entertainment sector. Even though they both use hypnosis, the end goal and the context are completely different.

12 Week Hypnotherapy Program

The most effective product we found for reducing weight was a 12-week hypnotherapy program.

The program does take some commitment as each of the hypnosis recordings have been split right into twelve sessions, among which needs to be listened to daily.

Week 1

In the first week of the hypnotic course, you are provided with the foundations for your brand-new weight management regimen.

Along with setting a weight-loss target on your own, you are additionally skillfully guided to eliminate a lot of your self-imposed restricting ideas surrounding your capability to produce and maintain a healthy and balanced, non-fat, and fit body.

Week 2

In the second component of the course, you learn precisely how to determine your body's all-natural signals. If you are starving, your body lets you recognize it!

When you are full, your body allows you to know! You will learn just how to identify between a desire and what to consume.

When you additionally use hypnotherapy to get over this emotional belief of what to eat, you will make sure that your daily consumption of food is significantly minimized.

Week 3

Neuro-Linguistic Programming (NLP) is used to change your mental patterns and practices. NLP is a highly effective and scientifically confirmed collection of strategies made to create immediate behavioral changes.

When used along with hypnosis, NLP ensures that behavioral adjustment is rapid advertisement long-term.

Week 4

Making use of hypnotic sessions to direct your memory back to the primary source of your over-eating, then removes the causes leaving you without emotional consumption.

Week 5

In week five, you are emotionally conditioned to drink a lot of water. Because it loads you up, water is an excellent help in weight loss.

Water intake reduces cravings pangs. It also has terrific lots of health and wellness advantages and gets rid of contaminants from the body.

Week 6

In these sessions, you are conditioned to incorporate light, natural exercise right into your everyday regimen to enhance your metabolic rate and slim down faster.

Hypnotherapy can be a significant help in any weight-loss program and has been revealed to generate some incredible results very quickly. Weight loss through hypnosis is not a "magic tablet."

It becomes compelling when combined with a physical weight loss regimen or diet regimen and exercise program. Water is a fantastic help in weight loss since it fills you up.

Week 7

At this point in the training course, you are conditioned to begin eating more healthily.

Week 8

This is designed to help you raise your metabolic price by gaining straight access to your subconscious mind and changing the plan it holds for your body.

Although, as we stated earlier, many other hypnotic CDs try this method, it functions in this course because you have already been conditioned to take more workouts!

The hypnotic ideas used during this week will help you get even more out of your exercise regimen and hence burn fat quicker!

Week 9

As you move closer throughout the hypnotic weight loss course, you will surely make use of the Swish method to ensure that the brand-new practices you have discovered come to be irreversible.

Week 10

Currently, it's time to make use of your subconscious mind's power to help you burn much fatter. Through the effective hypnotic pointers, you can command your subconscious mind to consume more of the kept fat in your body.

The training course will actively transform your consuming habits and exercise level even more!

Week 11

This week deals with the essential issue of self-image! Ensuring you have a positive self-image and a healthy and balanced respect for your body will ensure you stay healthy and balanced and do not abuse your brand-new ability to drop weight!

Week 12

Week 12 coatings your program. You ought to currently be seeing major arise from the work you have previously done. You are provided with recommendations that enhance your new practices and maintain you motivated to maintain a healthy and balanced fit body.

Using hypnotherapy as a quick-fix option for your weight issues will not work! Using it as a tool to aid you in shedding weight might well be the difference between success and failure. If you absolutely and truthfully choose to shed weight and establish a healthy and balanced body, hypnosis is most definitely a way to make the essential modifications easy, long-term, and rapid.

The program is a behavioral-change system made to assist you to attain your perfect weight and make that adjustment irreversible. Because it alters your behavior and attitude to food and exercise, at the subconscious degree, once you end up the course, it just really feels all-natural for you to preserve your brand-new healthy and balanced overview and practices to consuming and workout!

CHAPTER 8:

How to stay motivated

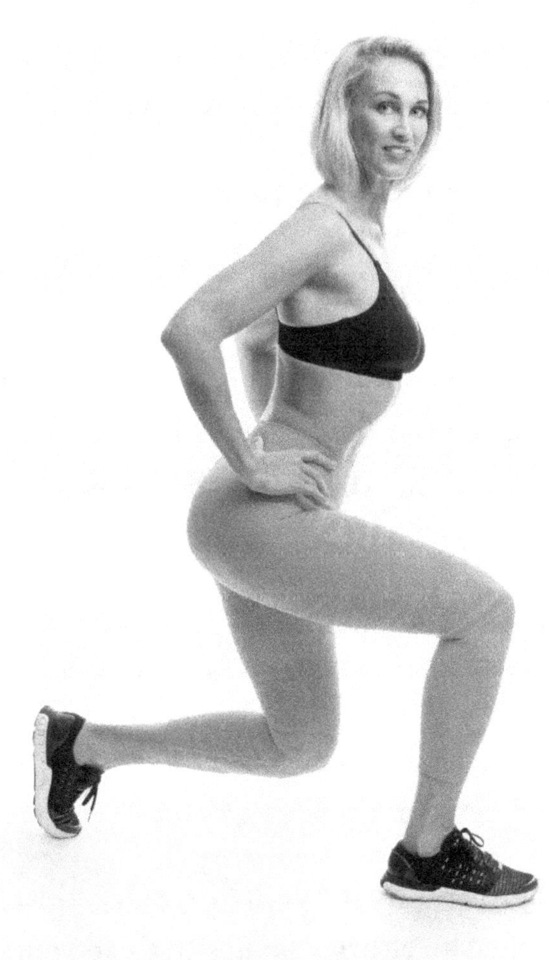

Motivation is one of the most powerful tools in creating permanent change. Your motivation is based on what you believe. And as you are probably aware, belief is scarcely based on your concrete reality. In essence, you believe things because of how you see them, feel them, hear them, smell them, and so forth. You can program your mind by taking feelings from one of your experiences and connecting those feelings to a different experience. Let us look at how you can remain motivated to lose weight:

Establish where you are now

You should take a full-length picture of yourself at present as a push mechanism from your current position. Two primary factors are relevant to health. One is whether you like the image you see in the mirror and the second is how you feel. Do you have the energy to do what you wish, and are you feeling strong enough?

Explore your reasons for wanting to lose weight. These are what will keep you going even when you don't feel like it.

Assess your eating habits and establish your reasons for overeating or indulging in the wrong foods.

It is assumed that you have the desire to get healthier and lose weight. Here, you state clearly and positively to yourself what you want, and then decide that you will accomplish it with persistence. Use the self-hypnosis routine explained above to drive this point into your subconscious mind.

Determine your motivation for the desired results, and how you will know when you've accomplished the goal. How will you feel, what you will see, and what are you likely to hear when you achieve your goal.

Devote the first session of self-hypnosis to making the ultimate decision about your weight. Note that you must never have any doubt in your mind about your challenge to lose weight.

Plan your meals every day. Weigh yourself frequently to monitor your progress as well. However, do not be paranoid about weighing yourself as this can actually negatively affect your progress.

Repeat to yourself every day that you are getting to your ideal weight, that you've developed new, sensible eating habits, and that you are no longer prone to temptation.

Think positively and provide positive affirmations in your self-induced hypnotic state.

Tweak Your Lifestyle

Every little thing counts. This is an important thing to note if you want to lose weight and slim down. Making a few changes in your regular daily activities can help you burn more calories.

Walk more

Use the stairs instead of the escalator or elevator if you're just going up or down a floor or two.

Park your car a mile away from your destination and walk the rest of the way. You can also walk briskly to burn more calories.

During your rest day, make it more active by taking your dog for a long walk in the park.

If you need to travel a few blocks, save gas and avoid traffic by walking. For greater distances, dust off that old bike and pedal your way to your destination.

Watch how and what you eat

A big breakfast kicks your body into hyper-metabolism mode so you should not skip the first meal of the day.

Brushing after a meal signals your brain that you've finished eating, making you crave less until your next scheduled meal.

If you need to get food from a restaurant, make your order to-go so you won't get tempted by their other offerings.

Plan your meals for the week, so you can count how many calories you are consuming in a day.

Make quick, healthy meals so you save time. There are thousands of recipes out there. Do some research?

Eat at a table, not in your car. Drive-thru food is almost always greasy and full of unhealthy carbohydrates.

Put more leaves, like arugula and alfalfa sprouts on your meals to give you more fiber and make you eat less.

Order the smallest meal size if you really need to eat fast food.

Start your meal with a vegetable salad. Dip the salad into the dressing instead of pouring it on.

For a midnight snack, munch on protein bars or just drink a glass of skim milk.

Eat before you go to the grocery to keep yourself from being tempted by food items that you don't really plan to buy.

Clean out your pantry by taking out food items that won't help you with your fitness goals.

The whole idea in the tweaks mentioned is that you should eat less and move more. You may be able to think of additional tweaks. List them down together with the ones found in this book.

Motivational Affirmation

Motivational affirmations are phrases, sentences, or even words that will enable you to stay positive, be focused, and be highly motivated. You need to choose these affirmations and use them on your daily basis. They are of great help as they will help you to meditate correctly on your weight loss. You can only reduce weight when you stay focused and positive. Being true to yourself and getting motivated every time will enable you to be able to control your weight. Even though these affirmations are numerous, you need to take a look at the ones I have detailed or illustrated the most common ones in the below paragraphs. It is good to note that, these affirmations, you can use each morning after just waking up. They will sincerely help you to jump-start your day on a much higher note. It is a challenge thrown at you that you better try this and see how your life will drastically change. Your mindset will shift, and you will only be thinking positively. You will only be staying focused on your life, and this will increase your esteem within and outside your external world. Below are some of the examples that you need to go through with much keenness.

You must embrace success. In every kind of situation or no matter the condition you are facing, tell yourself about success. You need to talk about being successful every morning. The word "you can't" should not appear in your mind. Everyone has excuses. Some excuses emerge from the fear of not trying. You need to stay focus and embrace the successful part of you. Don't get overwhelmed and overtaken by negative thinking about your success story. I challenge you to recite this affirmation every time you wake up. You will realize how important it is not only to your body but also in your external world. You need to feel unstoppable and fail to look at your excuses for not being successful. Negativity here is a BIG NO for you.

You must always be calm when faced with conflict. Conflicts are issues that always take you back to where you were. Conflict will automatically kill your daily morale leading to weak contributions of your abilities, especially within the organization and other sectors of life. You must try as quickly as possible to brush off annoyances easily. You must always agree with all sorts of disagreements so that the argument can end there. Tell yourself that you are more significant than what you are facing, and this should not drain you physically. Staying focused with a fit body and soul will make you lead a positive life.

At last, your weight will be highly controlled. You need to have that habit of doing this any time you are facing any conflict. It will only help you to stay positive and highly productive under your capacity. Reciting this affirmation every morning will be of great help. Try it as many as possible and help yourself to stay calm, relaxed, and comfortable.

You must choose to show love and gratitude every day. You need to know that life is always short and concentrating on negativity is not good. It won't go well with you. It will only derail your success. After all these, you must radiate elements of joy to yourself and have that love of your body. Showing all kinds of gratitude will enable you to lead a happy life. It will affect not only you but also the people around you. You must embrace this no matter what happens. Staying scorned and having negative thoughts only ages you as quickly as possible and leaves you with a body shape you never wanted. Be happy always and show love to the surrounding. You must try this and believe me, and you will have a change within the next few weeks.

You must be impressive to others. Staying positive in life is an excellent deal for yourself. Use anything under your disposal to impress those who are around you. You need to be positive in everything to be as positive as you can and never underrate yourself. No one sent a letter to be born in a certain way, so you need to accept yourself the way you are. It will enable you to stay focus and lead a real-life every day. You need to develop this habit of saying this affirmation to yourself as it is of great help. It will also help you to start your day with big morale and a notch higher.

You are free to develop your reality. Realities are things that are with us no matter what happens. Therefore, you must strive hard to create your reality. No one is supposed to create you one since you are in a better position with much knowledge about yourself. You must have a choice and choose wisely in every kind of situation you might get yourself herein. Remember, nothing should stand in between you and your happiness peak. That apex of goodness should be your cup of joy, and no one should prevent you from creating this form of reality for you. Choosing your reality every day will make you stay positive and entirely focused on life. Besides, it will be of great help as far as your body is concerned. Remember to note that your life ultimately depends on the realities within you. You can lie to people around you, but believe me, and you cannot lie to yourself. Therefore, it will be of great advice that you keep this affirmation as it will help you live and stay positive. In the end, this will automatically reflect on your body shape and image.

You need to shed off any unimportant attachment. Unimportant attachments are things that no longer have any effect on your life. These are things that will only let you down, thus derailing your life goals of achieving a mind-set full of happiness. Your future success depends heavily on this, and for you to get at that position, you will need to detach yourself from anything that might let you down. You must note that anything might also mean any person. We have people in our lives that always try very hard to put us down. These types of people are afraid of your success in life. They will try their best to pull you down, no matter how hard you try to embrace only positivity in your life. It is time to get yourself going and void them like the plague. Remember, you must live and not only live but choose a pleasant experience. It will only be possible if you manage to refuse anything or anyone that is holding you back. Since I have said this, it is now my wish that you may practice this affirmation and use it as your routine daily. Practice makes perfect, and you will only realize that when you train.

You are enough just as you are. You must release that demonic notion of having comparisons between you and others. For you to stay specific, you must have some success standards. After developing all these, set your own goals and ambitions. Your vision should relate to your mission in life. After all these, you can now judge yourself using the basis of your success. Those rules and regulations you created in your success standards should enable you to judge yourself accordingly. Just know you are just enough the way you were born. You are a complete soul, and no part of you is lacking. So never try to make a comparison with others. You should note that affirmation helps in the realization of worthiness. Within a short period, you will be able to control your body image. Also, it will be of a great deal as it helps you in achieving some of the personal goals in life and having a sound body is one of them.

You must be in a position to fulfill your purpose. The world should know your existence, and you must be ready to show your achievement. Showing your accomplished goals will need some positive deeds that lead to a successful life. On most occasions, people who trend are our trendsetters. They trend because of having done something positive or negative. They are then known all over the world. However, in this motivational affirmation, you need to focus on positive things. You need to be a trendsetter in showing the whole world what you are capable of offering. If you have been employed somewhere to sweep, you must clean until the country president cuts short his journey to congratulate you. Achieving your best is always one decisive way to be successful and lead a happy life free from stress and distress. Remember, this affirmation reminds you that no one has that power to stop you from doing or rather fulfilling your purpose in life. Sharing this thought every morning when you wake up will eventually get you somewhere. You must now stay focus and have this habit of telling yourself that no one can prevent you from achieving.

You must be results-oriented. In your daily life, you need to stay focus in life. Your primary focus should be on your results. It is through this that you will be able to realize your productivity.

To achieve this, you must be able to create some space for success. Get more success in your life. Avoid any derailing excuses that will only demean your reputation, thus lowering your success rate. Offer yourself these phrases every morning, and you will be in great joy for the rest of the day. You need not hold on to excuses for failing to achieve something. Be yourself and have the ability to struggle until you reach that success in life. It is through this that your mind will have settled, giving you peace of mind. Peace of mind will enable you to lead a stress-free experience. It will reflect in your body image.

Be in control of your won happiness. Happiness is an aspect of life that will initiate your feelings and moods towards a positive experience. It is like a gear geared towards your prosperous life. Staying positive here will be of great importance, and for you to realize this, you must take control of your happiness. Responsibility is a virtue and being responsible will make you bold enough to face all kinds of situations. Your joy is your key to success, and no one should tamper with it. Make happiness your priority and be responsible for it. You must let no one make you angry. Angriness will only induce you with emotional feelings that will eventually affect your life more so your body image. Having seen this, you must now be in an excellent position to embrace this affirmation. Take it as an opener to your morning and employ it entirely in your life.

CHAPTER 9:

The power of affirmations

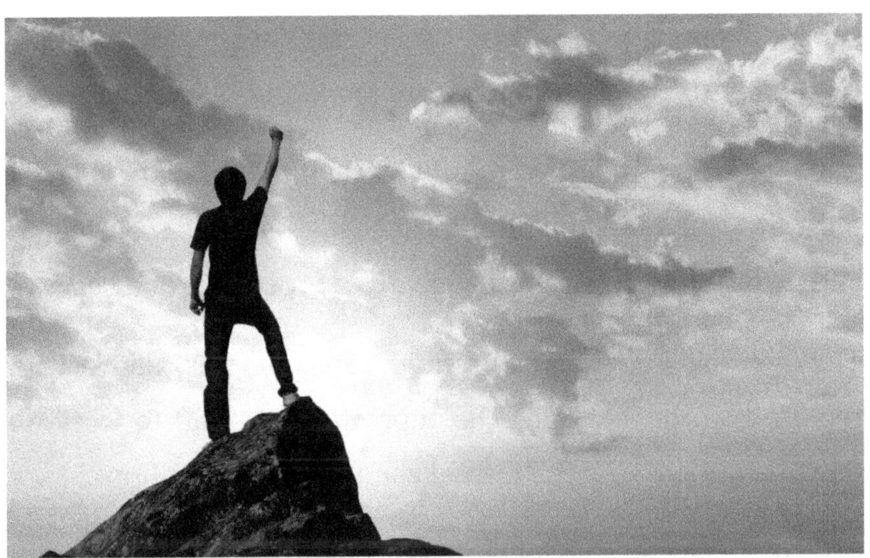

What Are Affirmations and the Way Do They Work?

Positive affirmations are positive statements describing a desired outcome, routine, or goal you wish to achieve. Repeating these positive statements often affects the subconscious mind deeply, and stimulates it into action, bringing into real life what you are parroting.

The act of mentally or loudly repeating the affirmations motivates the individual to repeat them, enhances confidence and inspiration, and creates incentives for change and success.

This act also programs the mind to act in accordance with repeated words, sparking the subconscious mind to work on one's behalf, making the factual claims come to fruition.

Affirmations are really helpful in creating healthy routines, achieving meaningful improvements in one's life, and attaining goals.

The affirmations help to lose weight, to become more centered, to learn more, to improve behaviors, and to fulfill goals.

They may be useful in athletics, industry, health-enhancing, bodybuilding, and many other fields.

These positive statements affect the body, the mind and one's feelings in a favorable way

It is very normal to repeat affirmations, but most individuals are not conscious of this. People often echo pessimistic, not constructive proclamations. This is known as negative self-talk.

When you tell yourself how miserable you are, how inadequate to learn, have not enough resources, or how tough life is, you reinforced pessimistic affirmations.

In this way, you generate more difficulties and many more issues because you focus on the troubles, and therefore increase them, rather than concentrating on the solutions.

Most people repeat negative words and statements in their minds about the unpleasant experiences and situations in life and thus create more unwanted situations.

Anytime you repeat something to yourself aloud, or in your thoughts, you're affirming something to yourself. We use affirmations consistently, whether we consciously know it or not. For instance, if you're on your weight loss journey and you repeat "I am never getting to lose the weight" to yourself daily, you're affirming to yourself that you only are never getting to succeed with weight loss. Likewise, if you're consistently saying, "I will always be fat" or "I am never getting to reach my goals," you're affirming those things to yourself, too.

When we use affirmations unintentionally, we frequently find ourselves using statements that will be hurtful and harmful to our psyche and our reality.

You might end up locking into becoming a mental bully toward yourself as you consistently repeat things to yourself that are unkind and even downright mean. As you are doing this, you affirm a lower sense of self-confidence, a scarcity of motivation, and a commitment to a body shape and wellness journey that you simply don't want to take care of.

Affirmations, whether positive or negative, conscious, or unconscious, are always creating or reinforcing the function of your brain and mindset.

Each time you repeat something to yourself, your subconscious hears it and strives to form a neighborhood of your reality. This fact is often because your subconscious is liable for creating your truth and your sense of identity.

It creates both around your affirmations since these are what you perceive as being your absolute truth; therefore, they create a "concrete" foundation for your reality and identity to rest on.

If you would like to vary these two aspects of yourself and your experience, you're getting to got to change what you're routinely repeating to yourself so that you're not creating a reality and identity rooted in negativity.

To vary your subconscious experience, you would like to consciously choose positive affirmations and repeat them continuingly to assist you in achieving the truth and identity that you only genuinely want.

This way, you're more likely to make an experience that reflects what you're trying to find, instead of an experience that reflects what your conscious and subconscious have automatically picked abreast of.

The key with affirmations is that you simply got to understand that your brain doesn't care if you're creating them intentionally or not.

It also doesn't care if you're creating healthy and positive ones or unhealthy and negative ones.

All your subconscious cares about is what's repeated thereto, and what you perceive as being your absolute truth.

It is up to you and your conscious mind to acknowledge that negative and unhealthy affirmations will hold you back, prevent you from experiencing positive experiences in life, and end in you feeling incapable and unmotivated.

Alternatively, consciously choosing healthy and positive affirmations will assist you with creating a healthier mindset and an identity that serves your wellbeing on a mental, physical, emotional, and spiritual level. From there, your responsibility is to repeat these affirmations to yourself until you think them consistently, and you start to ascertain them being reflected in your reality.

The only thing that is important when it comes to health and fitness is a balanced bodyweight. What decides your health is your weight! That's why, any time you go for a checkup, doctors always check your weight. The problem today is that people do not look at weight loss as a health problem anymore, instead of considering it as more of a looks problem, which is why they don't get anywhere. If they could only understand how important weight is to health, people would be more inspired to lose weight.

Your weight makes you who you really are. Whether you like it or not, you will be judged by it; this is just part of life. In fact, in America alone, over 65% of the population is either overweight or obese. That's two out of every three Americans. There are over 1 billion individuals worldwide that fall into this group! That's 1 in every 7 people around the world who have weight issues! It's no wonder healthcare is such a big issue.

So, you need to lose weight quickly and lose it right away, whether you're overweight or obese, but how are you going to lose weight the best way? The response to that is the biggest hidden weight loss mystery. The basic fact is that individuals DON'T know how to lose weight. In hopes that it will succeed, many will only try the old eat less and exercise more theory. Nonetheless, this mentality of weight loss is what ultimately keeps the world the same way with the same issues. People only do whatever the media and so-called experts tell them while doing the little operation. This is because there is no balance, which is why many struggle to lose weight!

The key to weight loss is balance. Every day, you need to eat the correct number of calories and exercise for the correct amount of time each week. For overall and long-term results, getting the balance is the best way! It's so important to understand because the secret of equilibrium can go to such endless depths.

However, you need to be well informed about it and its relationship with weight loss to make use of balance. You need to learn more about weight loss and all the elements of it. If you're serious about weight loss, then you can spend some of your time learning the secrets of weight loss. It's not going to be that hard if you know what there is to know about it.

If you want to really go further into weight loss, you're going to find there's so much more to it. Many factors have to be considered, including a good diet, weight, metabolism, and even the human body itself! In order to grasp weight loss entirely, there are so many things to remember.

You must first become educated about weight loss if you really want to commit to it. You need to get to the point where you will be able to spot it immediately if you make a mistake, without any support from experts or professionals. To succeed, you need to be totally alone.

Positive words are strong words that we repeat (either in our mind or out loud) to ourselves, and they are usually things we want to do. They are used to stimulate our inner thoughts and to affect our behavior and the progress we make. If you say them frequently with confidence and true conviction, then your subconscious mind will come to recognize them as genuine. Your new positive self-image will be improved, and you will be charged with positive energy. Your mindset, actions, and thoughts will shift and bring about a positive change until your mind begins to believe something is real. Positive remarks can be customized to any purpose you want to reach, including losing weight.

Try to use optimistic phrases that work for you and that you feel comfortable with. You have to repeat them regularly (at least 3-4 times a day) and with real certainty in order for them to work. Repeat them when you wake up in the morning and the last thing before you go to bed. Saying them out loud can be very motivational if you can get time alone. Write down your optimistic affirmations on a card and bring them around with you for an immediate boost at any time. You might also be able to post them on your fridge, a brilliant way to make you think twice about unhealthy snacks.

How's your loss of weight going? Are you losing the weight you thought you were going to lose? The expectations we set for losing weight often do not necessarily align with the actual act of losing weight. It can be really tempting to feel like it's pointless at times such as this, to just forget it and give up, then go back to the old way of eating.

In addition to keeping, you on track with your weight loss goals, optimistic words can be incredibly helpful by inspiring you to stay on this healthy track every day.

Affirmations and visualizations are tools that are used to accomplish almost anything in life, and there is no exception when it comes to weight loss. If that is so, why do so many people insist that statements don't work?

They need to be carried out properly in order for them to work. Some individuals feel that they can master a specific subject simply by seeking knowledge here and there. Quite often, in order to achieve success, a mastery of the subject is necessary.

The mediocre life that individuals build for themselves because of their negative thinking is a clear example of statements at work. Poor thinking plays a part in daily comments.

Note, it's not easy to do. Negative thinking is a custom, and it takes a deliberate, persistent effort to break a habit.

How to Use Affirmations and Visualizations for Successful Weight

Rule 1: never use phrases that are negative. Affirmations are directed towards the subconscious mind, and negative phrases are not defined by the subconscious mind. For instance, if you say "I am no longer overweight", the subconscious mind focuses on the "overweight" aspect and ensures that you stay overweight because it sees it as something you want.

Rule 2: using the claims only in the present tense. Do not say, "With this program, I will lose weight"; instead say, "I weigh 120 pounds right now" (if your target weight is 120 pounds).

Rule 3: be insistent. Don't give up ever. Everything you have now in your life is because of years of poor thinking. It will take some time before you begin to see good things about your life, but often you will be shocked by how easily things can change.

What keeps you from reaching your weight loss target? There may be several causes and explanations, such as medicine or disease, to blame for difficulty losing unnecessary pounds.

A hormonal imbalance can interfere with weight gain fluctuations. Emotional tension and adverse thoughts can dampen your spirits and send conflicting messages to your body. Just like your goals, a negative body image and attitude may also cause your body to respond.

Using helpful weight loss tips and motivation will set you on a healthy path, while melting fat cells to balance your body and mind.

Learning Affirmations is an Essential Step to a Slimmer You.

It could be said that there are literally dozens of proven and effective ways of programming your subconscious mind for weight loss hypnosis. However, out of all the hypnosis for weight loss techniques, none have the lasting power and motivating effect of positive affirmations. Why? Because it's a basic skill for lifelong success as your new slimmer self, well worth the time it takes to learn the skill, including how to write and use your affirmations, how to integrate them into your daily routine, and how to add them to your regular exercise. This article will explain how to use affirmations with hypnosis for weight loss.

It can take months for some clients to fully learn hypnosis for weight loss. I spent four weeks with Colin "under my wing". He studied some of the most effective personal enhancement techniques, and he studied almost all the tight-lipped secrets that weight loss hypnosis has to offer. However, once he began using three basic sentences, each day in three different settings, that was when he realized the improvements had taken place.

A basic formula for using affirmations and weight loss hypnosis is available. On an index card, you write down each and every one of your optimistic affirmations. Each day, you can take out a new card and re-affirm your statement. You can only start up again when you get to the end of the cards. You could have as few as three cards, or one for every day of the year. It comes down to whatever works for you best. The following are some examples of affirmations.

When it comes to affirmations, everyone is special, but here are the top three that I found with Colin. When you practice hypnosis for weight loss, you will find that you have your own favorites. "Day by day, I am getting slimmer and slimmer in every way." This is an old affirmation that has been around for years and has a compounding impact on the subconscious mind when properly repeated. "I am happy, safe, prosperous, and smart" and "I now have everything I need for permanent weight loss". Use these three affirmations as a start, and you can build ones that work for you with practice. Use them as follows.

In different settings, you may want to use these optimistic affirmations at least three times per day, including when you work out and before you go to sleep at night. You could even incorporate them into your morning walk to work. One instance is to say something when you work out, like "I have a fantastic body" and "I love my body". You are programming yourself with optimistic thinking, good emotions, and new habits that will affect you, even though you don't believe that this is valid. These new affirmations will soon become your normal way of thinking and repeating them over and over again will create a condition of self-fulfillment for you. You set yourself up to win.

In order to make your change last, it will take some engagement and constant effort on your part. So, make sure to learn and use these sample affirmations and produce your own weight loss script hypnosis. Do the exercises and compose and add your own affirmations that relate to you into your everyday life. The drug has been prescribed to you, and now it's your turn to take it.

How Do I Pick and Use Affirmations for Weight Loss?

Choosing affirmations for your weight loss journey requires you first to understand what it's that you are merely trying to find, and what sorts of positive thoughts are getting to assist you in getting there. You'll start by identifying what your dream is, what you would like your ideal body to seem and desire, and the way you would like to feel as you achieve your thought of losing weight. Once you've got identified what your idea is, you would like to spot what current beliefs you've got around the hope that you simply are meaning to achieve.

For example, if you would like to lose 25 pounds so that you'll have a healthier weight, but you think that it'll be incredibly hard to lose that weight, then you recognize that your current beliefs are that losing weight is tough. You would like to spot every single opinion surrounding your weight loss goals and understand which of them are negative or are limiting and preventing you from achieving your goal of losing weight.

After you've got identified which of your beliefs are negative and unhelpful, you'll choose affirmations that are getting to assist you in changing your beliefs. Typically, you would like to settle on a statement that's getting to help you completely change that belief within the other way.

For example, if you think that "losing weight is tough," then your new affirmation might be "I lose the load effortlessly." Albeit you are doing not believe this further affirmation immediately, the goal is to repeat it to yourself enough that it becomes a neighborhood of your identity and, inevitably, your reality. This way, you're anchoring in your hypnosis sessions, and you're effectively rewiring your brain in between sessions, too.

As you employ affirmations to assist you achieve weight loss, I encourage you to try to so in a way that's intuitive to your experience.

There are no right or wrong thanks to approaching affirmations, as long as you're using them daily. Once you are feeling yourself effortlessly believing in a statement, you'll start incorporating new affirmations into your routine so that you'll still use your affirmations to enhance your wellbeing overall. Ideally, you ought to always be using positive affirmations even after you've got seen the changes you desire, as statements are an exquisite thanks to naturally helping maintain your mental, emotional, and physical wellbeing.

What Should I Do with My Affirmations?

After you've got chosen what affirmations you would like to use and which of them are getting to feel best for you, you would like to understand what to try with them! The only thanks to using your affirmations are to select 1-2 statements and repeat them to yourself daily. You'll repeat them anytime you are feeling the necessity to re-affirm something to yourself; otherwise, you can repeat them continually, albeit they are doing not seem entirely relevant within the moment.

The keys to making sure that you simply are always repeating them to yourself so that you're more likely to possess success in rewiring your brain and achieving the new, healthier, and simpler beliefs that you got to improve the standard of your life.

In addition to repeating your affirmations to yourself, you'll also use them in many other ways. A method that folks like using statements are by writing them down.

You can write your affirmations down on little notes and leave them around your house; otherwise, you can make a ritual out of writing your statements down a particular number of times per day during a journal so that you're ready to work them into your day routinely. Some people also will meditate on their affirmations, meaning that they essentially meditate then repeat the affirmations to themselves over and over during a meditative state.

If repeating your affirmation to yourself sort of a mantra is just too challenging, you'll also say your chosen affirmations to yourself on a voice recording track then repeat them to yourself on loop while you meditate.

Other people will create recordings of themselves repeating several affirmations into their voice recorder then taking note of them on loop. At the same time, they compute, eat, drive to figure, or otherwise engage in an activity where affirmations could be useful.

If you want to form your affirmations productive and obtain the foremost out of them, you would like to seek out how to bombard your brain with this new information necessarily. The more effectively you'll do that, the more your subconscious mind goes to select abreast of it and still reinforce your new neural pathways with these new affirmations. Through that, you'll end up effortlessly and naturally believing within the new statements that you simply have chosen for yourself.

How Are Affirmations Going to Help Me Lose Weight?

Affirmations are getting to assist you in reducing during a few alternative ways. First and foremost, and doubtless most blatant, is that the indisputable fact that statements are arriving to help you get within the mindset of weight loss.

To put it simply: you can't sit around believing nothing goes to figure and expect things to think for you. You would like to be ready to cultivate a motivated mindset that permits you to make success. If you're unable to believe that it'll come true: trust that it'll not come true.

As your mindset improves, your subconscious is getting to start changing other things within your body, too.

For example, instead of creating desires and cravings for things that aren't healthy for you, your body will begin to make desires and cravings for items that are healthy for you. It'll also stop creating inner conflict around making the proper choices and taking care of yourself. You'll even end up falling crazy together with your new diet and your new exercise routine.

You will also likely end up naturally leaning toward behaviors and habits that are healthier for you without having to undertake so hard to make those habits. In many cases, you would possibly create practices that are healthy for you without even realizing that you simply are creating those habits.

Rather than having to consciously become conscious of the necessity for habits, then fixing the work to make them, your body and mind will naturally begin to acknowledge the need for better practices and can create those habits usually also.

Some studies have also suggested that using affirmations will help your brain and subconscious govern your body differently, too. For instance, you'll be ready to improve your body's ability to digest things and manage your weight naturally by using affirmations and hypnosis. In doing so, you'll be prepared to subconsciously adjust which hormones, chemicals, and enzymes are created within your body to assist with things like digestive functions, energy creation, and other weight- and health-related concerns that you may have.

You can use these affirmations as there; otherwise, you can adjust them to match what you would like for your belief system. If you are doing rewrite them, confirm that you simply are creating ones that directly reflect what you would like to listen to so that you'll change your beliefs to ones that are more supportive and less limiting.

Words work to build or demolish in both ways. It is the manner we utilize them that decides how they can produce positive or negative outcomes.

Positive affirmations to help you get started

- I'm grateful that I woke up today. Thank you for making me happy today.

- Today is a very good day. I meet nice and helpful people, whom I treat kindly.

- Every new day is for me. I live to make myself feel good. Today I just pick good thoughts for myself.

- Something wonderful is happening to me today.

- I feel good.

- I am calm, energetic, and cheerful.

- My organs are healthy.

- I am satisfied and balanced.

- I live in peace and understanding with everyone.

- I listen to others with patience.

- In every situation, I find the good.

- I accept and respect myself and my fellow human beings.

- I trust myself; I trust my inner wisdom.

- Do you often scold yourself? Then repeat the following affirmations frequently:

- I forgive myself.

- I'm good to myself.

- I motivate myself over and over again.

- I'm doing my job well.

- I care about myself.

- I am doing my best.

- I am proud of myself for my achievements.

- I am aware that sometimes I have to pamper my soul.

- I remember that I did a great job this week.

- I deserved this small piece of candy.

- I let go of the feeling of guilt.

- I release the blame.

- Everyone is imperfect. I accept that I am too.

- If you feel pain when you choose to avoid delicious food, you need to motivate yourself with affirmations:

- I am motivated and persistent.

- I control my life and my weight.

- I'm ready to change my life.

- Changes make me feel better.

- I follow my diet with joy and cheerfulness.

- I am aware of my amazing capacities.

- I am grateful for my opportunities.

- Today I'm excited to start a new diet.

- I always keep in mind my goals.

- I imagine myself as slim and beautiful.

- Today I am happy to have the opportunity to do what I have long been postponing.

- I possess the energy and will to go through my diet.

- I prefer to lose weight instead of wasting time on momentary pleasures.

- Here you can find affirmations that help you to change serious convictions and blockages:

- I see my progress every day.

- I listen to my body's messages.

- I'm taking care of my health.

- I eat healthy food.

- I love who I am.

- I love how life supports me.

- A good parking space, coffee, conversation. It's all for me today.

- It feels good to be awake because I can live in peace, health, love.

- I'm grateful that I woke up. I take a deep breath of peace and tranquillity.

- I love my body. I love being served by me.

- I eat by tasting every flavor of the food.

- I am aware of the benefits of healthy food.

- I enjoy eating healthy food and being fitter every day.

- I feel energetic because I eat well.

- Many people are struggling with being overweight because they don't move enough. The very root of this issue can be a refusal to do exercises due to negative biases in our minds.

- We can overcome these beliefs by repeating the following affirmations:

- I like moving because it helps my body burn fat.

- Each time I exercise, I am getting closer to having a beautiful, tight shapely body.

- It's a very uplifting feeling of being able to climb up to 100 steps without stopping.

- It's easier to have an excellent quality of life if I move.

- I like the feeling of returning to my home tired but happy after a long winter walk.

- Physical exercises help me have a longer life.

- I am proud to have better fitness and agility.

- I feel happier thanks to the happiness hormone produced by exercise.

- I feel full thanks to the enzymes that produce a sense of fullness during physical exercises.

- I am aware even after exercise, my muscles continue to burn fat, and so I lose weight while resting.

- I feel more energetic after exercise.

- My goal is to lose weight. Therefore I exercise.

- I am motivated to exercise every day.

- I lose weight while I exercise.

- Now, I am going to give you a list of generic affirmations that you can build in your program:

- I'm glad I'm who I am.

- Today, I read articles and watch movies that make me feel positive about my diet progress.

- I love it when I'm happy.

- I take a deep breath and exhale my fears.

- Today I do not want to prove my truth, but I want to be happy.

- I am strong and healthy. I'm fine, and I'm getting better.

- I am happy today because whatever I do, I find joy in it.

- I pay attention to what I can become.

- I love myself and am helpful to others.

- I accept what I cannot change.

- I am happy that I can eat healthy food.

- I am happy that I have been changing my life with my new healthy lifestyle.

- Today I do not compare myself to others.

- I accept and support who I am and turn to me with love.

- Today I can do anything for my improvement.

- I'm fine. I'm happy for life. I love who I am. I'm strong and confident.

- I am calm and satisfied.

- Today is perfect for me to exercise and to be healthy.

- I have decided to lose weight, and I am strong enough to follow my will.

- I love myself, so I want to lose weight.

- I am proud of myself because I follow my diet program.

- I see how much stronger I am.

- I know that I can do it.

- It is not my past, but my present that defines me.

- I am grateful for my life.

- I am grateful for my body because it collaborates well with me.

- Eating healthy foods supports me in getting the best nutrients I need to be in the best shape.

- I eat only healthy foods, and I avoid processed foods.

- I can achieve my weight loss goals.

- All cells in my body are fit and healthy, and so am I.

- I enjoy staying healthy and sustaining my ideal weight.

- I feel that my body is losing weight right now.

- I care about my body by exercising every day.

CHAPTER 10:

Increases your self-esteem every day

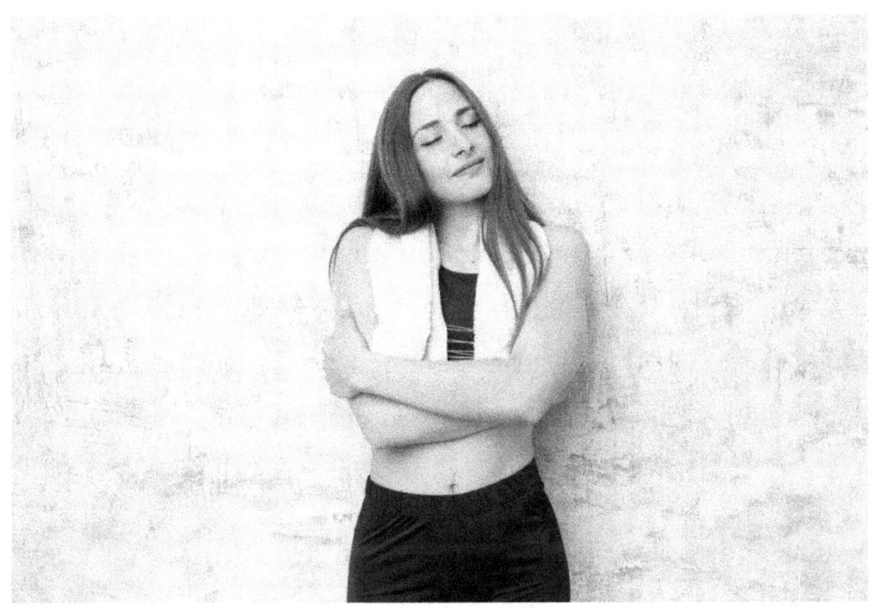

There's Self-Esteem, Then There's Confidence

You might be thinking that self-esteem and self-confidence are the same things--and many people do use those terms interchangeably--but there is a significant difference between the two. Self-esteem refers to how you value yourself. This is often based on social norms, and you frequently measure yourself in comparison to other people. For example, you might think, "I'm as intelligent and attractive as the next guy. Sure, I'm not a supermodel, but I'm not chopped liver either." Or, you might think, "I wish I were as witty as she is. I can't think of things to say as fast as most people can." Both of these statements reflect a valuation of yourself in comparison to other people.

If you have high self-esteem, you are comfortable in your skin. You're happy with who you are, regardless of how you might measure up to the next person. You can recognize and appreciate the gifts that other people might have, but this is important--you also acknowledge your contributions. You know that the offerings of other people do not detract from those of your own. You understand that you don't have to have the same gifts that everyone else has.

If you have low self-esteem, on the other hand, you will continuously not measure up, which can lead to depression and a sense of hopelessness. It can cause you not even to try because you think you will never succeed. You will also likely be submissive to other people's wishes because you don't believe you can lead the way, even if we're talking about your own life. Additionally, you'll often find yourself feeling guilty as if you have done something wrong when, in fact, you've done nothing to be guilty about. You might think you have to prove you're as good as someone else, and for that reason, you likely will set an unrealistically high standard for perfection. That sets you up for failure, which reinforces the low opinion you already have of yourself. It's a vicious cycle. But you might be thinking that you do have confidence in your ability to get things done. Ah, but confidence is a horse of a different color.

Self-confidence is how we view our ability to do something, like overcome an obstacle or improve a skill. It's really about how you perceive your ability to get the job done. While it is true that completing tasks successfully can increase your self-confidence, and that can, in turn, increase your self-esteem, it is also possible that you can have high confidence and low self-esteem. You can believe that you can get the job done and simultaneously think you're not the right person.

On the other hand, you can have high self-esteem and low self-confidence. You can value yourself as a person but question your ability to do the job. This might be exemplified by people you know with high self-esteem who are extremely competent at a particular task (or even many tasks), but who are continually questioning their work. They double and triple check themselves with every job they do. It's not that they think they're not intelligent enough to do the job, but they question their ability to get it done correctly. They always fear they will make a mistake. This is low self-confidence in action.

On the other end of the spectrum, people with high self-confidence can easily cross the line into arrogance. We tend to admire confident people, but what makes them sure is that they don't feel the need to advertise their skills. They know they have done the job well or have a particular talent, and they don't have to show off those skills to prove themselves. When people feel the need to flaunt their abilities, this is referred to as arrogance. In reality, it's another type of confidence, a false bravado that people project to cover what is likely their low self-esteem. These are the loud, opinionated, and often abrasive people in the presentation of their views. If someone feels the need to pander for adoration or is continuously looking to demonstrate they are the most knowledgeable or most capable individual, it likely indicates they secretly have a low opinion of themselves and seek external approval to prop up their self-image.

At this point, you might also be wondering about humility. Isn't being humble a good thing? Humility is defined as having a modest view of one's importance. But this doesn't mean exactly what it sounds like. It is not encouraging low self-esteem. Instead, there is a difference between how you value yourself as a person and how you view your contributions in life. For example, you can know you are the right person and that you contributed in a meaningful way to the successful completion of a project, but at the same time, you can know that it was a team effort that got the job done. You can also understand that the completion of the project is more important than any one person's contribution alone.

To sum it up, self-esteem is the value you place on yourself. Self-confidence is the view you have of your ability to get something done, and humility knows that, while you know you are valuable and capable, there are more important things than your accomplishments. Arrogance is when you feel the need to flaunt your abilities or achievements, and it often masks low self-esteem. But how do these things form? When do we develop our image of ourselves and our belief, or lack thereof, in our abilities?

The Impact of Social Media on Self-Esteem and Confidence

One of the problems with social media is that people tend to share only their highlights, which creates an image of constant happiness that might not reflect reality. It creates an unrealistic appearance with which you might be comparing yourself. It appears all your 'friends' are always enjoying life and experiencing success, and you feel like you're not measuring up.

But that's not reality. What you're not seeing is the behind the scenes struggles that they also go through as they face numerous challenges. They post that they got a new job, and you think, "Wow! How easy that was for them, and now they're off on a new, exciting adventure." However, what they didn't post were the numerous applications and perhaps some failed job interviews that came before they finally got the new job. You don't see the self-doubt they experienced about whether they would be able to find a new job. Also, it might not just be your friends' profiles that depress you. You might become depressed by your profile if you realize that your posting is an illusion. You might think you're not living up to your own best self.

Does this mean you have to stop using social media? Maybe! It would be best if you took whatever means are necessary to prioritize building up your self-esteem and confidence. Perhaps it doesn't mean you have to stop using social media but consider taking a break from it while you focus on yourself if you feel it is holding you back. Whatever you decide to do, you need to realize that what you see on social media is the best face put forward by your many friends. It's like pictures in a photo album; you don't see the sad moments or the depressing and challenging times. You see the happy times, the successes, and the smiles. But, it's just a moment in someone's life, and it's usually just the best moments that they take a picture of, and then post on social media. That doesn't mean they don't have bad moments too--they're just not posting those in the same way you are likely not posting your fears, anxieties, and difficulties in life. As with your 'physical' friends, you should seek out positive virtual friends and get rid of any virtual friends trying to tear you down. Virtual bullying can be even more damaging than what happens on the school playground since you can at least escape the playground. Be careful about who you "friend" --make sure they're someone who will appreciate you! Remember, all the rules of building your self-esteem and self-confidence apply to the virtual realm as well as the physical.

Managing the Media Impact on Self-Esteem for Healthy and Sustainable Weight Loss

What does your body resemble? The odds are that you have at any rate a couple of flaws that stress you and keep you from tolerating and cherishing your body.

As indicated by a 2014 report, almost 10 million ladies in the UK experience uneasiness and sorrow in light of their looks. One in every four ladies has avoided getting a charge out of a personal connection on account of her appearance. Almost 25 percent of the ladies examined detailed that stresses regarding appearance have kept them from seeking after work.

What's considerably more problematic - 36 percent of the ladies addressed said that they don't practice as a result of stresses over appearance and being taunted at the exercise center.

Media set inconceivable magnificence and wellness principles. By far most ladies would never draw near to those unreachable pictures of flawlessness.

Unimaginable self-perception depiction is additionally holding up the traffic of effective weight reduction by influencing self-discernment and fearlessness.

The Media Influence on Body Image

Media have sway on all ladies - from youthful and naive adolescents to senior women. One thing is sure - we don't appear as though big names and the exceptionally controlled pictures cause individuals to feel totally lacking in their skin.

Magazines, films, music clasps and sites all present unreasonable flawlessness. Obviously, a great deal of this flawlessness originates from picture handling, yet the photos are amazingly incredible and powerful.

Being fit and solid is adjusted to being thin, a condition that is unsafe yet that an ever-increasing number of individuals are beginning to grasp.

Positive Body Image for Successful Weight Loss

Effective and reasonable weight reduction ought to be about wellbeing instead of unreachable excellence beliefs. It requires a difference in attitude, which can be especially hard to achieve. Contrasting ourselves with others is an ordinary piece of human instinct and breaking out of the awful media cycle requires cognizant exertion and quality.

Investigate you - what number of models do you see strolling around? Customary ladies have bends, cellulite, stretch imprints, dull spots and different flaws. It's urgent to comprehend that you're contrasting yourself with something that doesn't exist.

Affirmations for Self-Esteem

When it involves body image, self-esteem is vital. Low self-esteem is often both the explanation for an undesirable body image and, therefore, the results of one. If you are unhappy with how you look and feel, it might be because you lack the vanity to form a change; otherwise, you may feel that way due to how your health is within the times.

Either way, boosting your self-esteem can now help keep you committed to your wellness goals and may improve your ability to foster a body shape and level of health that feels more desirable for you.

- I deserve a happy, healthy life and body.

- I'm a singular individual.

- Life is fun and rewarding.

- I need to have a body that helps me explore everything that life has got to offer.

- I select to be happy and healthy immediately. I like my life.

- I select to possess a pleasant experience.

- I really like and accept myself as I'm.

- I'm thriving now and forever.

- Every day I take a step toward becoming my best self.

- I need to love my body.

CHAPTER 11:

How to Use Meditation and Affirmations to Lose Weight

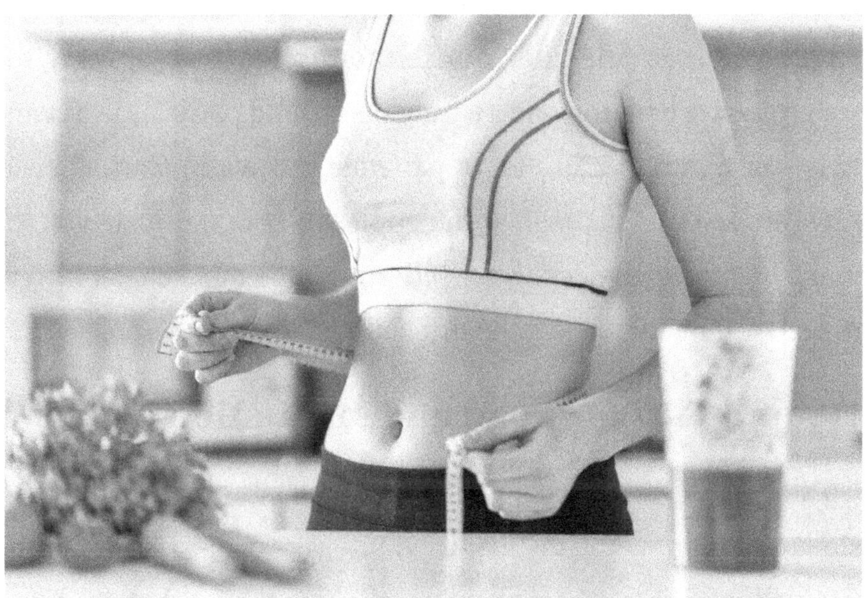

People always associate bodyweight genes or external factors like, eating habits, available food at one's disposal, or emotional stress. People do try to escape the fact that they are responsible for their eating choices and the quantity of the food they eat. This makes it easy to go back to our original poor eating habits even after we have started meditation. However, through meditation, we get to understand our role and contribution to our own journey to weight loss. Changing one's eating habits and patterns is not an easy step and requires a lot of patience, motivation, and focus. Always surround yourself with people who can motivate you to make healthier choices. We need not blame our genes but try to work on making better health choices.

Helpful Tips for Food and Meditation

Go slow with your meals, put more emphasis on chewing very slowly, and know the taste of each bite. Treat the moment as if you will describe to someone exactly how the food tastes like. By doing this, it helps you keep the focus on the food you eat and appreciate different taste, even the most unpleasant.

Create a mealtime and adhere to it. Avoid eating when you are doing something else; also, this prevents overindulging and helps you measure the quantity as well as eat to satisfaction and not leisure. Multitasking, as you eat, can lead to overeating or indulging in unhealthy foods.

Respond to hunger and satisfaction. When you are hungry eat do not deny your body food, this also applies to when you are full; you should stop eating. Listen and communicate with your body whatever it is telling you to respond appropriately.

Know how different kinds of food make you feel. This is after you eat them. This statement mostly responds to questions like, which meal makes you tired or energized? Avoid food that makes you tired since they reduce the body's metabolism.

Learn to forgive yourself for overindulging even when you are not hungry. The food that you ate because you wanted to but made you tired just forget about them and continue with the food that keeps you energized. Understand that you are not perfect and are bound to be tempted to eat the foods you don't want to eat. When you give in to temptation, forgive yourself, and move on.

Spend time and make responsible food choices, always plan for the kind of foods you'll eat in advance. If you can't do this all the time, make a weekly or daily meal plan.

Acknowledge your food cravings. By doing this, you will be able to resist your craving by understanding that it is reasonable to crave, but you do not have to give in to all types of cravings.

We can design specific techniques and practices concerning mindful eating, meditating, and intuitive eating. By these techniques, we get to have a healthy and productive relationship with regards to food and thereby to eliminate any bad feelings associated with diet and our eating habits. The result of this is healthy weight loss though this should not be the key focus; it should serve more as a reward. If we focus on weight loss as the primary goal, then we may be distracted and not have a focused mind during meditation. When eating, though, you should eat because you are hungry and need to satisfy yourself. Do not eat because you are stressed at work, stressed with family issues, so you need to eat to forget about your stress. Meditation practices help you love your body and be in control of your mind and the decisions you make.

General Health Affirmation

They are statements, phrases, or words that you use in your daily life. Their main task is to give you that maximum motivation in everything that you do. Remember, you always speak these words to yourself. Phrases like this include;

"I can radiate confidence." Confidence refers to the ability to show boldness in what you are doing. You must now be in a position to radiate not only faith but also grace and beauty. Virtues like these are highly significant since they will always guide you daily. You will feel relaxed, motivated, and have the urge to be successful in life. Your health improves, and you will be able to see this in your body image. Elements of grace and beauty will affirm you to your real-life situations. You will be able to maintain this kind of morale, which will eventually help you to make correct decisions on your healthy food. It is good to state that choosing a healthy diet is not only useful to your life but also economical. A proper diet, too, results in an accelerated appetite and urge even to eat more. Healthy food is always good for your body as it supplies you with enough nutrients. Nutrients have the power of smoldering your body, thus improving your body image.

"Every cell within my body accepts good health." You must ascertain yourself always with these words. Good health will always make your whole body vibrates. It is now up to you to concentrate on maintaining good health throughout. You can do this by choosing healthy food from the stores. Healthy eating includes plant-based diets that have less content of meat. The healthy meal plan also incorporates a large intake of water, daily exercises, and eating healthy. All these nourish your body cells, making them carry out their work accordingly. Your motivation to eat every day will develop suddenly, especially when you have all these healthy food at your doorstep. In the long-run period, your body weight reduces due to the assimilation of a healthy diet. Fortunately, in the end, your body image improves, leading to shedding off some pounds.

You must love and show some respect for your body. Your body is built up with so much complexity that when you fail to prove it, love, you can even fail. Show some love to your body by providing everything that it needs.

The body needs nourishment, which comes from food. Choose as healthy as possible food. Healthy food will offer your body that glimmering natural look. You will also reduce weight, thus improving your body image. Elements of love, respect, and other virtues always act as stimuli that help you to achieve much in your body. You will realize that your weight reduces without facing difficulties in the process. Reduction in weight will come as a result of choosing wisely the correct diet and using an affirmation to accelerate their intake in your body. Another general health affirmation is to be in a situation where you can choose issues like health and wellness, and shun or shy off boring workouts, restrictive diets, and so on. I know you might love workouts, but some exercises are just unpleasant. Instead of helping you get over your weight, they will load you with exhaustion, bruises, and other minor injuries. Again, there are restrictive diets that you need to shy off. Eating meat-related meals, completely processed flour, and relying much on junk dishes will only affect you negatively. It is because of this that you choose your body health and its wellness. You can improve your body health by deciding on a healthy diet. Your welfare, too, is paramount. It matters a lot not only to you but also to your general economic status. Making these choices will accelerate your need to have healthy food at your disposal. As a result, your motivation to eat healthy increases a notch higher. All these will lead to improved body image with a decrease in your weight.

Transcendental Meditation and Weight Loss

Meditation is generally utilized as an unwinding instrument, similar to a back rub for the psyche. What's more, much the same as there are numerous approaches to create an organic product serving of mixed greens; meditation accompanies an assortment of systems. One specific sort called Transcendental Meditation (TM) has earned the distinction since the 1960s after a celebrated musical crew called "The Beatles" began rehearsing it.

Here are the means to rehearse TM:

- Take a seat, assuming a comfortable position. Do not cross your arms or legs.

- Make sure your eyes are closed. Take several deep breaths to bring the body into relaxation.

- Open your eyes shut them once more. Your eyes will assume this state for the whole 20-minute duration.

- Decide on the mantra to recite in your mind.

- When you notice that the mind has started to wander, refocus your attention back to the mantra.

- After the whole duration is over, slowly move your toes and fingers to return you to reality.

- Open your eyes.

- If you do not feel prepared to go on with your day, sit for a longer duration.

- Indeed, you might think about how TM will help with weight decrease. As per research directed on veterans experiencing PTSD, when the psyche rises above, the body comes into an expression far more profound than even profound rest and goes there undeniably more rapidly. Stress prompts a characteristic instrument, which is intended for our assurance to endure.

This pressure logically triggers various exercises to counter the response:

- The front piece of the cerebrum will be detached, the part which is liable for drive control.

- The creation of the bliss hormone "dopamine" diminishes (the pressure hormone "cortisol" increments.

- Individuals under pressure are less and less able to tune in to the reasonable needs of the body.

Rising above is fundamentally the contrary experience of pressure, and that way, it will have the opposite impacts. The subsequent harmony enables the body likewise to increase exceptionally profound rest (further than rest), in which it can disintegrate even its most profound anxieties aggregated because of life's most exceedingly terrible injuries. As we develop revived and renewed from the quietness of meditation, this can deliver different emotional upgrades in any part of our life.

Mindful Eating

We eat mindlessly. The principal explanation behind our awkwardness with nourishment and eating is that we have overlooked how to be available. Careful eating is the act of developing a receptive familiarity with how the food we eat influences one's body, sentiments, brain, and all around us. The training improves our comprehension of what to eat, how to eat, the amount to eat, and why we eat what we eat. When eating carefully, we are entirely present and relish each chomp - connecting every one of our faculties to value the nourishment. Past simple tastes, we see the appearance, sounds, scents, and surfaces of our food, just as our mind's reaction to these perceptions.

Steps to Mindful Eating

Watch Your Shopping List

Shopping mindfully, – purchasing sound nourishments that are reasonably delivered and bundled – is a significant piece of the training.

One thing you will probably find about careful eating is that entire nourishments are more dynamic and heavenly than you may have given them acknowledgment for.

Learn How to Eat Slower

Eating gradually does not need to mean taking it to limits. It is a smart thought to remind yourself, and your family, that eating is not a race.

Setting aside the effort to relish and make the most of your nourishment is perhaps the most advantageous thing you can do. You are bound to see when you are full, you'll bite your food more and consequently digest it all the more effectively, and you'll likely end up seeing flavors you may find some way, or another have missed.

Eat When Necessary

However, it might take some training to locate that sweet spot between being eager and hungry to the point that you need to breathe in a dinner.

Additionally, tune in to your body and get familiar with the distinction between being physically eager and sincerely ravenous. On the off chance that you skip dinners, you might be so anxious to get anything in your stomach that your first need fills the void instead of making the most of your nourishment.

Enjoy Your Senses

The vast majority partner eating with simple taste and many eat so carelessly that even the taste buds get quick work. Be that as it may, eating is a blessing to a higher number of faculties than simply taste. When you are cooking, serving, and eating your nourishment, be mindful of shading, surface, fragrance, and even the sounds various nourishments make as you set them up. As you bite your food, take a stab at distinguishing every one of the fixings, particularly seasonings. Eat with your fingers to give your feeling of touch some good times. By drawing in various faculties, the entire experience turns out to be significantly more completely fulfilling.

Keep off Distractions

Our day by day lives are brimming with interruptions, and it is normal for families to eat with the TV boom or one relative or another tinkering with their iPhone. Think about making family supper time, which should be eaten together, a hardware-free zone. This does not mean eating alone peacefully; careful eating can be a tremendous mutual encounter. It just means you do not eat before the TV, while driving, on the PC, on your telephone, and so on. Eating before the TV is the national hobby, however, simply consider how effectively it empowers mindless eating.

Stop when you are full

The issue with astounding nourishment is that it tends to be challenging to quit eating by its very nature. Eating gradually will enable you to feel full before overeating. Still, on the other hand, it is imperative to be mindful of segment size and tune in to your body for when it starts disclosing to you it has had enough. Gorging may feel great at the time; however, it is awkward for a short time and is commonly not beneficial for the body.

Meditating to Heal Your Relationship With Food

The capacity to hold a full scope of various feelings for the day is a test for a considerable lot of us. We simply need to feel upbeat, yet the test is to locate that mystical parity of all that we experience, decipher, and do. The most natural history of past weight reduction endeavors is ceaseless confinements, which requires self-discipline and force. This perspective has a negative turn and does not draw out the best of us.

Mindful Eating Meditation Script

Start by interfacing with your breath and body, feel your feet on the ground, and notice your involvement at this time. With your mindfulness at this time, see any contemplations, sensations, or, then again, feelings you are encountering.

Tune into the mindfulness or impression that you have in your collection of inclination eager, parched, or perhaps feeling full. On the off chance that you would eat or drink something at present, what is your body hungry for? What is it eager for? Simply focus and notice with mindfulness the vibes that give you this data. (Interruption)

Presently, get your regard for the thing in your hand and envision that you see it just because. See with interest as you focus and notice the shading, shape, surface, and size. Is there something else that you notice, sense, or feel? (Interruption)

You are allowed to alter the procedure just as you would prefer.

Utilizing a care-eating exercise is just a single piece of a caring way to deal with your eating regimen. The freeing intensity of care produces further results when you start to give careful consideration to your contemplations, feelings, and real sensations, all of which lead us to eat. Attention (mindfulness) is the establishment that numerous individuals have been missing for defeating nourishment longings, addictive eating, voraciously consuming food, enthusiastic eating, and stress eating.

Foods to Eat for Deeper Meditation

Meditation can be extreme. Take out every single stray idea? Concentrate just on your breath? Sit still for (at least) 10 minutes one after another? In any case, we are increasingly finding out that rehearsing everyday meditation has such a large number of astonishing advantages, from helping us become progressively empathetic to empowering us to be increasingly quiet, adoring, happy, excusing, and liberal.

Green Tea

Numerous old societies related to Tea with long life and wellbeing. Starting in China, it has been utilized as medication for a great many years. Green Tea has not exclusively been filling our mugs for quite a while yet has played a job as a fundamental fixing in numerous a sweet.

It has been the subject in various therapeutic and logical investigations to decide if it is since quite a while ago, toted medical advantages convey any legitimacy.

Tomatoes

A lot of vitamin C, which is generally viewed as valuable in bringing down your pressure. As per an investigation led in Japan, members who ate tomatoes over six times each week had an essentially lower danger of framing discouragement.

Specialists are attempting to make sense of whether lycopene, the synthetic segment that makes tomatoes dark red, legitimately influences psychological prosperity.

Lemon or Lemon Water

Lemons are generally plentiful in nutrients and minerals, especially nutrient C, a cell reinforcement that lifts the resistant framework, ensures against cardiovascular sickness, and helps avert malignant growth. Lemons likewise animate vitality and can help upgrade your state of mind. How? The two lemons and limes are one of only a handful couple of nourishments that contain more negative charged particles than positive ones, which gives your body an increase in vitality when it enters your stomach-related tract.

Nuts

Brimming with cell reinforcement Vitamin E and zinc, nuts, such as almonds, pistachios, and pecans, are useful for boosting the insusceptible framework. They likewise contain a lot of B-Vitamins, which help you oversee pressure and sadness. Scientists have demonstrated that nuts improve our cerebrums' capacity to tackle issues, one more significant piece of meditation.

Vegetables and Whole Fruits

Eating an eating regimen wealthy in whole foods grown from the ground is probably the best thing you can accomplish for your body. The equivalent is similarly valid for the brain. Root vegetables, including sweet potatoes, squash, and carrots, are pressed with a wide range of nutrients and minerals.

CHAPTER 12:

How to Practice Every Day

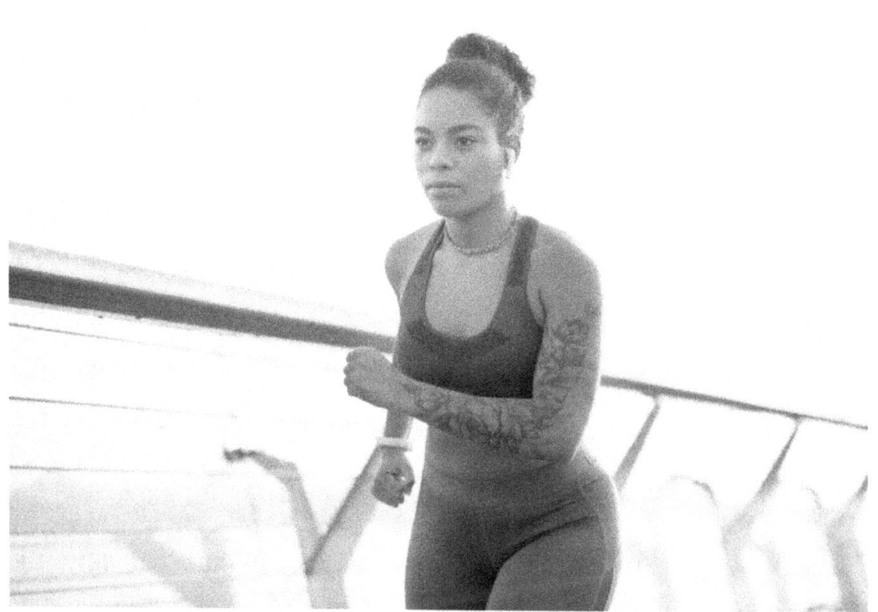

What is the secret to getting rid of weight problems? I am going to tell you. The trick is breaking the old subconscious blocks, generating new patterns of thought and harmonizing the conscious and subconscious mind. Hypnosis will help you conquer the subconscious bloc obstacles.

You'll feel better. They're going to feel in control. You'll feel sure to be able to control your weight with encouragement and determination to keep up with your weight loss goals. Hypnosis has none of the negative or harmful side effects of diet pills or surgery. If you choose a successful diet and exercise plan and then reprogram your mind to make it no longer challenging but simple, pleasant and efficient to follow your food and fitness programmer, you will certainly succeed.

Have fun exercising and eating healthy, so you can stop causing self-induced tension, stress and discouragement. You will start doing the things that will help you in your aim of being safe and losing weight, obviously. You need to get rid of the unhealthy habits of thought that make you overweight. These thought patterns, which are stored in your subconscious mind, must be replaced with healthier thoughts and healthy behaviors so that you can instinctively do what you are expected to do without ever thinking twice about it.

Does that sound tricky? In reality it's much less complicated than you would imagine. All you need is 10 to 20 minutes a day for a total of 21 days (the amount of time it takes to build a habit).

You can now have what it takes to speedily program your mind to lose weight. You see, hypnosis is one of today's world's most overlooked and powerful methods for self-change.

When you say "hypnosis," most people think of magic shows in Vegas or stupid acts on stage. Those on stage were chosen especially because of their susceptibility to suggestion. They wouldn't do anything that they normally wouldn't do on stage. For the publicity they receive, they really "do not mind" behaving stupidly on stage. If they don't perform, they know they're going to be taken off the stage and back to the seat. There could not be anything further from the facts. In theory, hypnosis is a very comfortable state of mind in which you become more receptive to suggestions. During the day, you usually go through hypnosis many times.

If the use of hypnosis for treating illness has been accepted by major medical societies, imagine how amazingly successful and beneficial it is when coping with thought patterns that stand in the way of the healthy body you deserve. The use of hypnosis has been used for more than half a century to treat illness. In addition, in 1955 the British Medical Association approved the hypnotherapy use. Its use was approved in 1958 by the American Medical Association.

In a 9-week trial-weight management group study (one using hypnosis and one not using it), the hypnosis group has continued to get results in the two-year follow-up, while the non-hypnosis group did not show any further results (Journal of Clinical Psychology, 1985). The groups using hypnosis lost an average of 16 pounds in a sample of 60 participants, while the other group lost an average of just 0.5 pounds (Journal of Consulting & Clinical Psychology, 1986). Multiple studies showed that the addition of hypnosis increased the weight loss by an average of 97% during treatment and, more importantly, the efficacy increased by more than 146% after treatment. Hypnosis is known to perform much better over time (Journal of Consulting & Clinical Psychology, 1996). "The best way to break bad habits is by hypnosis," even Newsweek Magazine said.

Whether you want to use audio tapes or CD's for hypnosis, review the script used to determine if the suggestions make sense to you. Make sure there are no suggestions that are negative.

The subconscious will not hear "no" or "no" so the suggestion 's emphasis would be: I do not consume fattening foods. This will give you your objective in the opposite direction. Just use constructive feedback. "I just eat fresh foods that make me feel solid, safe and happy" is much better.

When you get up in the morning and before going to bed in the evening is the best time for your mind to accept these positive suggestions. You need a quiet room where nothing won't bother you. When you're getting a lot of action in your house, you may need to find a room where you can shut the door and get undisturbed. It only lasts for 10 to 20 minutes.

Hypnosis is not a one-time fix for most people. The Hypnosis results are cumulative. The more post-hypnotic suggestions are applied to the hypnosis, the more permanent the results become. So, few people are likely to get hypnotized once to avoid smoking or lose weight. We usually create a new habit if they do, to replace the one they just quit. Most people who quit smoking begin overeating. We were replacing only one undesirable habit with another. Unless the root(s) of the problem is found there would be no need to add another habit.

Having a specialist skilled in hypnosis and weight loss struggles could prove useful. Working with a specialist will help you understand the earlier programming and remove it.

Especially with weight loss, use relaxation and self-hypnosis every morning and evening to be effective, changing and perfecting your suggestions while you lose weight. Upon reaching the weight you are comfortable with; you might want to add other goals along with strengthening your healthy eating and exercising habits.

You will need to start with the full relaxation at first, but after a week or so you will be able to go very quickly into the altered relaxed state by counting down from 10 to 1. Always end your session with a suggestion that makes you feel good, better than ever, relaxed and either alert, clear-headed, refreshed and full of morning energy or relaxed and able to sleep soundly when you go to bed at night.

Keep a pen and paper close by to write down any insights that come to mind while listening to your suggestions or reading them. You can recall things that you were told as a child that now influence your behavior.

CHAPTER 13:

Love your Body

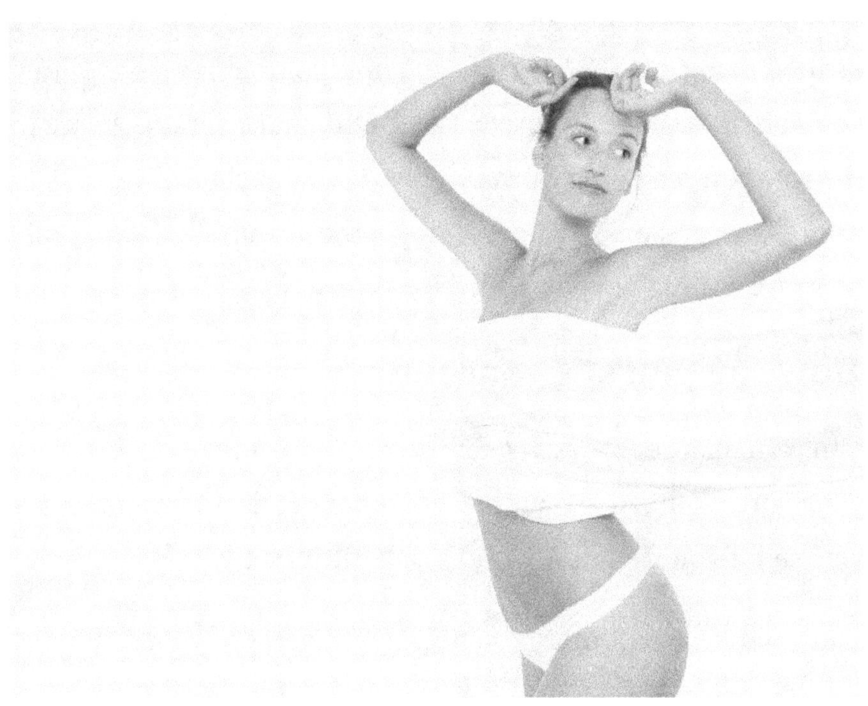

The majority of individuals don't think very much about self-improvement. We'd love to assist you to indulge in such a notion and find out just how much you can enjoy yourself. It's a requirement for accepting and creating your ideal weight and everything else that's fantastic for you. Just being conscious of the idea of self-help can move you farther along on the way of enjoying yourself and accepting yourself as you are. Your character and character are aware of the way you're feeling on your own. If you harbor bitterness or remorse, or sense undeserving, these emotions operate contrary to enjoying yourself.

How can you see your flaws?

Can you blame yourself? Self-love and finding an error or depriving yourself repaint each other. It is tough to enjoy yourself if you frequently find errors ultimately.

Can you pay attention to the negative aspects of yourself?

Can you end up making self-deprecating statements, such as "I am not intelligent enough to..." or even "I am not great enough to..."?

Can you punish yourself or refuse yourself?

Can you establish boundaries with individuals who represent your very own moral and ethical criteria and your values and beliefs?

Look at the mirror. How do you feel about yourself? Can you smile or frown?

Which are you about the continuum of self?

Are you currently respectful and admiring?

Are you critical and judgmental, or would you love yourself for who you are?

Have you been caring and caring for this individual who you see?

If you're ambivalent, then contemplate these concerns further. Be truthful with yourself. Have a conversation on your own. Take a sincere look at yourself. Do not just examine your own body; examine your wisdom, your soul, your own emotions, along with your own heart. Know that: By enjoying yourself, you love yourself. If there's something that you can't accept on your own, be aware you could change that idea, and alter it to make anything you want, such as your ideal weight.

The power of self-love and forgiveness

Have a Look at These characteristics? Are these familiar to you? It is the way it will feel for those who like yourself:

You genuinely feel happy and accepting your world, even though you might not agree with everything within it.

You're compassionate with your flaws or less-than-perfect behaviors, understanding that you're capable of improving and changing.

You mercifully love compliments and feel joyful inside.

You frankly see your flaws and softly accept them learn to alter them.

You accept all of the goodness that comes your way.

You honor the great qualities and the fantastic qualities of everybody around you.

You look at the mirror and smile

Many confound self-love with becoming arrogant and greedy. But some individuals are so caught up in themselves they make the tag of being egotistical and thinking just of these. We do not find that as a healthful indulgence, however, as a character that's not well balanced in enjoying love and loving others. It's not selfish to get things your way; however, it's egotistical to insist that everybody else can see them your way too. The Dalai Lama states, "If you do not enjoy yourself, then you can't love other people. You won't have the capacity to appreciate others. If you don't have any empathy on your own, then you aren't capable of developing empathy for others." Dr. Karl Menninger, a psychologist, states it this way: "Self-love isn't opposed to this love of different men and women. You cannot truly enjoy yourself and get yourself a favor with no people a favor, and vice versa." We're referring to the healthiest type of self-indulgence that simplifies the solution to accepting your best good.

Have a better look at the way you see your flaws and blame yourself. Self-love and finding an error or depriving yourself aren't in any way compatible. If you suppress or refuse to enjoy yourself, you're in danger of paying too much focus on your flaws that are a sort of self-loathing. You Don't Want to place focus on negative aspects of yourself, for holding these ideas in your mind, and You're giving them the psychological energy which brings that result or leaves it actual.

Self-hypnosis can help you use your mind-body to make new and much more loving ideas and beliefs on your own. It helps your mind-body create and take fluctuations in the patterns of feeling and thinking about what has been for you for quite a while, and which aren't helpful for you. The trancework about the sound incorporates many positive suggestions to change your ideas, emotions, and beliefs in alignment with your ideal weight.

Forgiving Yourself for Your Dietary Mistakes

Forgiveness is an underrated and essential element of weight loss. Often, people that are within the position of wanting or wanting to reduce and fail to acknowledge the very fact that they need been feeling incredibly frustrated with themselves. Anger, frustration, disappointment, and sadness directed at yourself once you are on this journey are all incredibly normal feelings to possess.

They can even be painful and overwhelming if you are doing not take the time to acknowledge them, forgive yourself, and heal them as you experience them.

You may end up feeling angry, frustrated, disappointed, or sad that you simply let yourself gain such a lot of weight. You'll fail to acknowledge the very fact that it had been not intentional, or that it had causes that were beyond your control, mainly if your weight gain was associated with medical conditions or a scarcity of education around healthy eating.

Regardless of what causes you to gain weight, you'll feel contempt for yourself for "allowing" it to happen, which may make it difficult for you to plan to lose weight.

When you sit in anger and frustration with yourself, it is often difficult to simply accept yourself as you're now and work toward improving your wellbeing through weight loss. Forgiving yourself for not knowing better or for not doing better, or maybe forgiving yourself for blaming yourself for something that was beyond your control, is vital.

The more you'll forgive yourself, the more likely you're to acknowledge that your weight is some things you would like to figure on. Through that, you'll be ready to work on weight loss from a peaceful frame of mind.

Studies have shown that those that accept themselves as they're and forgive their mistakes are more likely to lose the surplus weight and keep it off than those that refuse to forgive themselves. Refusing to forgive yourself can create a huge amount of stress inside you that creates it difficult for you to remain focused on exercising, eating healthy, and improving your wellness. Many of us find that this difficulty in forgiving ourselves worsens their self-esteem and self-confidence, which keeps them within the unhealthy cycle of behaviors and patterns that cause their weight gain in the first place. If you would like to beat these cycles, you would like to be willing to forgive yourself for your past choices, mistakes, and experiences which will or might not are beyond your control.

Another area where you would like to master forgiveness is within the process of change. As you progress faraway from old habits and behaviors and into a replacement way of taking care of your body, you're bound to make mistakes.

You are getting to have days or maybe weeks where you fall back to old patterns.

Some people even fall back to old patterns and stay trapped in them for years. This fact happens because they're unwilling to forgive themselves for creating an error, then they fall back to the cycle of contempt and low self-esteem and self-worth.

If you would like to be ready to continue moving forward together with your wellness and to leap back on target as quickly as possible, you would like to be willing to forgive yourself for any mistakes you create. This way means anytime you overeat, engage in an old eating pattern, choose an unhealthy food choice, or otherwise make a "mistake" in your diet, and you forgive yourself. Upon forgiving yourself, confirm that you also plan to take that have under consideration so that you'll make better choices. Make an honest effort to try to do better next time so that whenever you forgive yourself, you give yourself a reason to believe that your commitment to yourself genuinely means something. When you can forgive yourself and believe that your commitment to bettering yourself and your life means something, you start to create your self-esteem. Through that, things like portion control begin to become easier, and you discover yourself naturally gravitating toward taking better care of yourself.

How Does It Feel to Love Yourself?

Have a look at These features. Are these familiar to you? It is the way it should feel if you like yourself:

You genuinely feel happy and accepting your world, even though you might not agree with everything within it.

You're compassionate with your flaws or less-than-perfect behaviors, understanding that you're capable of improving and changing.

You mercifully love compliments and feel joyful inside.

You frankly see your flaws and softly accept them learn to alter them.

You accept all of the goodness that comes your way.

You honor the great qualities and the fantastic qualities of everybody around you.

You look at the mirror and smile (at least all the period).

Many confuse self-love with becoming arrogant and greedy. But some individuals are so caught up in themselves, they make the tag of being egotistical and thinking just of these. We do not find that as a healthful self-indulgent, however, as a character which isn't well balanced in enjoying itself love and loving others.

It isn't selfish to get things your way; however, it's egotistical to insist that everybody else can see them your way too. The Dalai Lama states, "If you do not enjoy yourself, then you can't love other people. You won't have the capacity to appreciate others. If you don't have any empathy on your own, then you aren't capable of developing empathy for others" Dr. Karl Menninger, a psychologist, states it this way: "Self-love isn't opposed to this love of different men and women. You can't truly enjoy yourself and get yourself a favor with no people a favor, and vice versa." We're referring to the healthiest type of self-indulgence that simplifies the solution to accepting your best good.

Just take a better look at the way you see your flaws and blame yourself. Self-love and finding an error or depriving yourself aren't in any way compatible. If you deny enjoying yourself, you're in danger of paying too much focus on your flaws that are a sort of self-loathing. You don't wish to place focus on negative aspects of yourself, for by keeping these ideas in your mind, you're giving them the psychological energy which brings that result or leaves it actual.

Self-love is positive energy. Blame, criticism, and faultfinding are energy. Self-hypnosis can help you utilize your mind-body to make new and much more loving ideas and beliefs on your own. It helps your mind-body create and take fluctuations in the patterns of feeling and thinking which have been for you for quite a while, and which aren't helpful for you. The trancework about the sound incorporates many positive suggestions to shift your ideas, emotions, and beliefs in alignment together with your ideal weight.

A Vital goal for all these positive hypnotic suggestions is the innermost feeling of enjoying yourself. If your self-loving feelings are constant with your ideal weight, then it is going to occur with increased ease. But if you harbor bitterness or remorse, or sense undeserving, these emotions operate contrary to enjoying yourself enough to think and take your ideal weight. Lucille Ball stated it well: "Love yourself first and everything falls in line" The hypnotic suggestions about the sound are directions for change led to the maximum "internal" degree of mind-body or unconscious. However, the "outer" changes in life action should also happen.

Many weight reduction methods you have been using might appear to be a lot of work. We suggest that by adopting a mindset that's without the psychological pressure related to "needing to," "bad or good," or even "simple or difficult," with no judgment in any way, the fluctuations could be joyous.

Yes, even joyous. It produces the whole journey of earning adjustments and shifting easier. The term "a labor of love" implies you enjoy doing this so much it isn't labor or responsibility. The "labor" of organizing a family feast in a vacation season, volunteering at a hospital or school, or even buying a gift for someone very particular can appear effortless. Here is the mindset that will assist you in following some weight loss methods. We invite you to place yourself in the situation of getting adored.

You're doing so to you. Loving yourself eliminates the job, and that means it is possible to relish your advancement toward a lifestyle that encourages your ideal weight. Think about some action that you like to perform. Imagine yourself performing this action today. Notice that whenever you're doing something which you love to perform, you're feeling energized and beautiful, and some other attempt comes out by enjoyment. What is going on at these times is you see it absolutely "loving what you're doing." Sometimes, we recommend that you also find that as "enjoying yourself doing this." Maybe by directing a more favorable attitude toward enjoying yourself, you'll end up enjoying what you're doing.

Conclusion

There are many reasons why someone should use hypnosis to lose weight. First, hypnosis is often successful when all other avenues of weight, health, and fitness have failed, and that's for a good reason!

The problem is not the method or even the plan you are using to achieve it. The problem is in your mind. If you want to lose real body fat, reduce weight, make your ideal shape, and maintain your new look, it is essential to change your attitude towards food and exercise, and your behavior towards both.

The best hypnosis programs for weight loss may require you to understand and replicate those mental processes used by people who have lost weight already. It might be tough leaving your comfort zone, but hypnosis will help you to reprogram your mind and install new thoughts that will become automatic habits once you identify the right behavior perfect for achieving your goal.

Eating less and adequately, or exercise following a schedule won't be a dream anymore: hypnosis enhances and strengthens your will.

So, if you are worried about being overweight now, there is nothing wrong with undergoing hypnosis. After all, you have nothing to lose

Ultimately, hypnosis, both in a professional or home setting, has the potential to help with weight loss. According to Vanderbilt University, hypnosis works best for individuals who need to lose low-to-moderate amounts of weight.

It doesn't mean that you shouldn't attempt it but talk with your doctor about working it into a routine that incorporates other weight loss behaviors. It requires a various number of hypnosis sessions by a hypnotherapist. It may take a long time before professional therapy alters your attitudes and actions, and it may take a while before changed behaviors become a habit.

Try not to get discouraged with little change. If nothing else, regular hypnosis sessions may help ease pressure and help you learn to relax, reducing your need to eat in emotional situations. Because hypnosis is probably not going to deal with the issue all by itself, consider keeping a food and exercise journal.

Also, record how long you practiced and what kind of activity you did. This log considers you accountable for poor decisions and allows you to distinguish patterns in your eating and exercise habits that may counteract healthy weight loss. When you identify these patterns, you'll have a venturing off point for your next hypnosis session, as far as critical thinking and behavior modifications may assist you with weight loss.

Regardless of how you approach hypnosis, its advantage may be what you have to finally lose that abundance of weight and carry on with a healthier life—good karma helps with using hypnosis to achieve your weight loss goals. Add up many small strides for weight loss success.

The more you practice the meditations we've given to you, the easier it will be to discover the success you've been waiting for. After a complicated diet, again and again, getting nowhere is an ideal opportunity to accept what isn't right about our mindset.

A perfect way to turn your mood around is to rework it through meditation. Tune in to these at whatever point you're home and find the opportunity. If you're exhausted, why not take a few minutes to relax and pull yourself together?

Whatever strategy for eating healthy you may pick; these meditations and trances will help you stop gorging and think it is easier to eat healthily and practice naturally. Recollect that it takes over one attempt and that you should practice it regularly, not once a month. When you can incorporate these snapshots of relaxation into your routine, it will help them work better.

All the best

www.ingramcontent.com/pod-product-compliance
Lightning Source LLC
Chambersburg PA
CBHW061754250726

48657CB00001B/123